Hot (Sweaty) Mamas

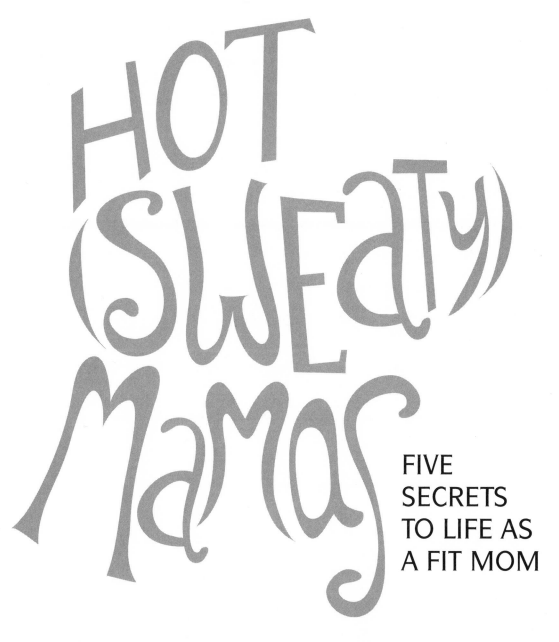

HOT
(SWEATY)
MAMAS

FIVE
SECRETS
TO LIFE AS
A FIT MOM

Kara Douglass Thom and Laurie Lethert Kocanda

Andrews McMeel
Publishing, LLC

Kansas City • Sydney • London

Andrews McMeel Publishing, LLC
an Andrews McMeel Universal company
1130 Walnut Street, Kansas City, Missouri 64106

www.andrewsmcmeel.com

Book design by Holly Ogden
Composition by Steve Brooker

11 12 13 14 RR4 10 9 8 7 6 5 4 3 2 1

ISBN: 978-1-4494-0245-7

Library of Congress Control Number: 2010930554

ATTENTION: SCHOOLS AND BUSINESSES

Andrews McMeel books are available at quantity discounts with bulk purchase for educational, business, or sales promotional use. For information, please e-mail the Andrews McMeel Publishing Special Sales Department: specialsales@amuniversal.com

For Tony, Cady, and Maggie.
Thanks for being my number-one cheering squad and support crew.
Once again, you've helped get me to the finish line.
—LLK

For Mark, McKenna, Kendall, Jocelyn, and Blake.
Thank you for inspiring me, motivating me, and cheering me on.
—KDT

Contents

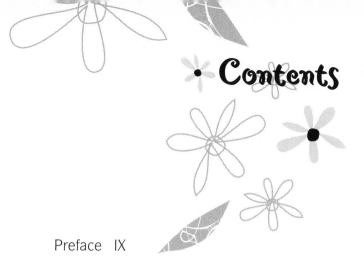

Secret Number Four

People Can Sabotage Your Fitness Faster Than A Cookie Binge . . . 113

Secret Number Five

Act Like Others Are Watching Because They Are . . . 139

You're a Hot (Sweaty) Mama Now . . . 177

Appendices . . . 180

The Conception of a Book

From Kara

Laurie and I met shortly after I moved to the Twin Cities from Texas in the summer of 2003. At the time, Laurie's daughter was a little over one, and my twins were newborns. We were both triathletes, writers who had read each other's bylines on occasion, and, now, moms. A couple of summers later, after the birth of my third daughter and Laurie's second daughter, we got together for lunch to hammer out a presentation for the Twin Cities Marathon Expo about managing fitness through pregnancy. I thought we made a good team since my prenatal fitness program slowed to leg lifts in the pool while Laurie was the sort to go for a run after her water broke—true story.

As we chewed on our sandwiches and discussed the outline for our talk, Laurie looked up and said, somewhat sarcastically, "Who cares whether or not you exercise during your pregnancy? The real challenge is finding a way to work out after the kids are born."

Talk about an "Aha!" moment. She nailed it, and yet, at the time, there was nothing out there that spoke to women about balancing fitness and motherhood. Plenty was said about fitness during pregnancy and ad nauseam about getting your body back after baby. (Insert eye rolling here, because none of those books adequately address how to get your body back after baby while said baby is clinging to your leg screaming, "Up! Up!").

When we parted ways after having lunch that day we had the beginning of an outline for a presentation as well as for a book.

From Laurie

Because we were living the life of *Hot (Sweaty) Mamas*, we had our own experiences, victories, and challenges to draw from for the book (even the title came to Kara in an indoor cycling class). This was good material, for sure, but we were just getting our legs as fit moms and it felt strange to be writing from a position of expertise. Four years later, with six kids between us, we're now comfortable with our expertise in this area. But the research and interviews with fellow fit moms that we did for this book also influenced the book (and us!) tremendously.

Still, I don't know that any of us feel that we've perfected the art of balancing motherhood and fitness. It's a constant effort, to be sure, but the outcome—a healthier, happier mom—is worth it. What's more, there's a funny little thing that happens as you make time in your life for exercise: Your kids watch. Our children are still quite young, so we don't have hard evidence yet that they will grow up to be active adults, but we are certain we are good role models for fit living and that our kids are more active now because of our lifestyle choices. *(They better grow up to be fit, or else!)*

Our Own History with Fitness

From Kara

My own fitness level was heavily influenced by fit family members. My mom was the first person ever to take me to a gym. I'm not sure how old I was—a tween, perhaps. We lifted weights together and my eyes bulged when I first noticed how cut my mom's arms were as she pulled the lat bar down. She also loved to ski and would escape on a Saturday alone, or with girlfriends, for a day trip to the southern New Mexico slopes. I never resented her for that "me time," and I look back fondly on her passion for speeding down a snowy mountain. My parents also played tennis, so I took lessons every summer, as well.

Then there was my uncle Bob, under whose guidance my family took active vacations before active vacations were hip. We went on family bike rides, rock-climbing trips, and hikes to Guadalupe Peak, the highest elevation in Texas. We even learned how to rappel off the flat face of a cliff in Hueco Tanks State Park. I spent much of my childhood and teen years dancing, as well, but once I graduated from college and I wasn't dancing regularly anymore, I needed to find another activity to keep me moving. Soon I found myself in a role I had never considered for myself: athlete. I became a runner and triathlete. I loved this outlet for my energy, what finish lines did for my confidence, and the social circles I was forming as a young adult (which would eventually lead me to my husband, Mark).

From Laurie

As the youngest of four children, I spent my childhood engaged in two-on-two games of football, hockey, and soccer. I ran the bases while my brothers played "hot box," even snagging a few blows to the head in the process. I spent countless hours swimming, biking, and hiking the wooded trails behind my home with my sister. In grade school, high school, and college, I played competitive team sports year-round, eventually feeling somewhat lost in the nonathletic world of adulthood. That's when I found my true passion for individual sports. After making my first trip to an indoor rock-climbing gym, I was hooked. I traveled around the country climbing anything I could get my hands on—both indoors and out.

Eventually, my focus shifted to running and I began training for my first marathon. Shortly thereafter, I met my husband, Tony, who also had a passion for fitness. Together we ran marathons in a number of different states, competed in adventure races and triathlons, mountain biked the trails of Moab, even ran from one rim of the Grand Canyon to the other and back. We got engaged on our first-ever kayak adventure. Before we started a family, we were each other's most frequent training partners, and our active lifestyle was something we were not willing to let go of. When people heard we were expecting our first child, they often told us we were in for a rude awakening. We were warned that we wouldn't have any time or energy left for working out, and that we should start looking for some new hobbies. Perhaps it was denial, but we ignored the comments and kept along with life as usual throughout both pregnancies. Setting a marathon goal after each delivery got me up and moving quickly after our daughters were born. It's taken some work, but we've managed to juggle life and keep our fitness routines going. We've proved those skeptics wrong.

The Birth of *Hot (Sweaty) Mamas*

From Kara

When I imagined myself becoming a mother, like many women pre-children, the reality was different from what I envisioned. When it came to my fitness, I expected to go on as usual. I expected to run through pregnancy—I even signed up for a 10K in my fifth month—and I visualized myself running with a jogging stroller and training and racing without any of the additional complications of motherhood (even though I didn't know what these complications might be). But early on I found I couldn't run like most of my pregnant runner friends. I took the assault to my ego but listened to my body. Good thing, because at my twenty-week sonogram we learned I was carrying twins. And, as any mom reading this book knows, there would be more hurdles to come.

As Laurie pointed out that day at lunch, it's great if women can exercise through their pregnancies, but it's only nine months. In the grand scheme of things, just a blip. What really matters is *Can you pick up the pieces and get back to fitness on less sleep than you thought was humanly possible?* "The uterus accommodates a baby better than a gym bag," Laurie wisely pointed out.

From Laurie

And so, over the course of four years, Kara and I carved out time to write, as well as work out, on top of the time we spent bringing income into the family coffers, being moms, keeping up with our homes, cars, dogs, and so on. We were our own lab rats as we attempted to nail down exactly what drove us—and other moms—to maintain our fitness in the midst of everything else we needed to do. We also went ahead and developed that presentation and have told the *Hot (Sweaty) Mamas* story to women at marathon expos and running stores, at mothers-of-multiples meetings and at church groups.

Without the input and perspectives of the many women we have met along the way and those who took the time to complete our survey, this book would not have as much depth or be as comprehensive as it is now. It's both amazing and endearing to know what moms will do to take care of themselves, to literally go that extra mile. We know there are many more women out there who want to join this community of *Hot (Sweaty) Mamas*. They might just need a little nudge in the right direction, some enlightenment to get going and keep going. Kara and I hope they find the motivation and some of the answers in these pages.

The Rise of the
Hot (Sweaty) Mama

Face it: As a mom, you're running around a lot, but you might not be logging many miles in your running shoes. Sometimes your daily responsibilities can be so hard to manage that the thought of throwing fitness into the mix is exhausting. "Just get me through today and I'll work out tomorrow." Right?

Perhaps you manage to fit in your workouts but are overcome with guilt when you think about the dozens of other "responsible" things you could be doing with your time. There are trade-offs for being fit; for instance, dishes pile up in the kitchen sink and your favorite bra goes AWOL in the mass of laundry breeding in the closet.

Being a mom isn't easy. But we love it. For most of us, raising children is our most meaningful experience in life. Why, then, does motherhood often leave us feeling tired, worn, and isolated? Perhaps even a smidge resentful over the body we're left with?

Think you're alone? Hardly. Hot (Sweaty) Mamas come in various shapes, sizes, and abilities. While we all have different experiences balancing motherhood and fitness, we do share a common goal: to enjoy a fit lifestyle that is part of our identity and that models healthy living habits for our kids. A mother's quest for fitness is the same, regardless of her fitness level. Balancing that juggling act between fitness and family is the common denominator between the likes of Dara Torres, Olympic swimmer, and the mom trying to get to the gym three times a week.

If you are inactive but ready to embrace fitness and make *fit mom* part of your identity, we'll spend some time in this book helping you make that leap—helping you come to the "other side."

Being on that "other side" may only be a state of mind. Some of us think of ourselves as fit moms, because we're convinced we'll get to that workout tomorrow. Still others may be committed to fitness but are left wondering if a good sweat is worth the hassle. In any case, we'll reconstruct your mental framework so that you not only fit fitness into your day but into your *life*.

No matter where you are now on this fitness journey, by book's end, you will be a Hot (Sweaty) Mama.

The Things Moms Do to Sweat

As we learned in our survey, some moms will go to extremes to find a way to work out. Are these good ideas or too crazy to consider? We're not endorsing or judging. Just saying . . .

- I made a four-by-six-foot box on the carpet with masking tape to exercise in, and told my girls they had to stay out of Mommy's box until I was done with my workout.
- Swung a kettlebell in the house, while children sat nearby watching Looney Tunes.
- Swam laps using a pull buoy between my ankles and dragging my daughter from it.
- Walked up and down the stairs in my house doing bicep curls with my two-month-old.
- Told my boss I had to leave early for a doctor's appointment so I could get a workout in before I had to pick up the baby from day care.
- Leaped up and down like a frog in front of the high chair. Yes, with ribbits. Try it! You will fell the burn!
- After forgetting my daughter's lunch box, I ran home and then ran back to school with it under my arm in order to get the first two miles of my run in.
- On a windy and rainy day I left both kids in the car watching movies on my iPhone while I did my CrossFit class in the park (with the kids in view).
- I once had to whip a nursing infant off a boob as the gun went off for a 5K. I started the run with her startled and half fed in a jog stroller!
- I ran up and down the stairs for thirty minutes. One child sat in a bouncy chair at the top of the stairs and the other sat with his blocks at the bottom of the stairs.
- Craziest thing I've ever "done" to get my workout in was *my husband* on our kitchen countertop. He never says no to me doing a long run after that!
- When I moved halfway across the country I packed the jogging stroller into my Honda Civic with everything else so I could run when we stopped for lunch every day.
- Pushed a double jogger with one hand that also had a dog leash wrapped around it while pulling a rope attached to a bike with a four-year-old novice cyclist.
- I've only been a mom for three and a half months, which hasn't really given me opportunity to do anything over the top yet. But I know my day is coming!

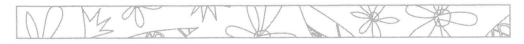

Your (Wonderfully) Complicated Life

Being a Hot (Sweaty) Mama offers a unique mix of complications. For starters, you don't have the luxury of working out whenever you like. Getting up early to go to the gym may not be an option if you're a single mom or if your spouse leaves for work at the crack of dawn. Postwork exercise isn't always feasible if your daughter has an evening basketball game or your son has a birthday party to attend (or if you're just plain spent from a long day). Even the best-planned workouts are in jeopardy of being replaced by a surprise visit to the doctor's office.

Whether you work outside the home or stay home to raise children is irrelevant. Both types of working mothers face fitness hurdles. If you have a career, time spent with the kids during the week can be hard to come by. Guilt does amazing things to moms, and it's no surprise that includes forgoing workouts to be with the children.

For stay-at-home moms, taking care of the kiddos for up to twelve hours at a stretch can create a deficit of time, energy, or both. And when you do find the time and/or energy to exercise, you may not always have the opportunity.

Almost every woman has some difficulty orchestrating her day to include fitness. Exercise programs designed to help new mothers return to "prebaby" shape are patronizing if they don't mention the logistics involved. Most of us don't have a grandparent living next door for impromptu babysitting. (If you do, you're the envy of most moms.) In theory, gym day care is great, but sometimes tears and germs do their best at keeping us away. Pushing two kids in a double jogger is a great cardiovascular workout . . . until the third baby comes along. Logistical nightmares can sully whatever motivation we have.

In addition to the demands of having children, you still have other relationships to tend to, including that with your spouse or partner. (Note: Throughout this book we'll refer to a spouse or partner as "he," though we know for some readers it should read "she.") There is the car to maintain (much more important when you're hauling precious cargo), the house to clean (an ever-elusive task once kids take over), coworkers to placate, and extended family to visit (now that you have children they want to see you). If you're a single parent, there is a whole different set of challenges for you to manage. There's no denying that life is more complicated; it's no wonder fitness often takes a backseat.

Some of us need a little kick in the behind to get us out the door each day, someone to tell us we need (and deserve) time to ourselves to become healthy in both body and soul. Others need help pulling in the reins and learning that it's OK to take a step back from working out—that our personal worth is not determined by times, miles logged, or a small waistline. The rest of us just might want reassurance or encouragement from this community of like-minded moms.

Welcome to life as a Hot (Sweaty) Mama.

As you may or may not know, the complications come with benefits of equal or greater value. Taking on these sorts of challenges ensures we take care of our health (like everyone says we should), maintain a sense of our self (easy to lose amid children's needs), and spread happiness into our home (happy mom, happy family—and we'll venture to say fit family, too).

The following are some of the issues Hot (Sweaty) Mamas face. We'll address them throughout the book as we help you successfully fold fitness into your daily life.

Identity Crisis

Even if you haven't been exercising (lately or ever), deep down inside you know there's a fit mama in there somewhere. And if you're new to fitness, we hope you identify with fit moms. Living a fit lifestyle starts with that vision of who you want to be.

Those of us who were fit before having kids shouldn't stop pursuing fitness goals after having children, just as we would never stop being a mom while breaking a sweat. They both are part of who we are.

MOM 2 MOM

I exercise because I feel like it is one of the last parts of prebaby me left. I love my kids but I feel like my identity was stolen when I had them. Running brings me back to me.

—Mechelle, mom of four
Chesaning, Michigan

The best way to gain or maintain that fit identity is to determine realistic fitness goals for yourself *at this stage in your life*—even if that's just committing to one workout a week. Maybe you were a competitive athlete before children—running road races most weekends in the summer. Or maybe you envision yourself at the top of your gym's climbing wall or mastering that kickboxing class. It doesn't matter. The first step is to decide what you want to do in this life of yours. What do you *want* to change and what do you *want* to stay the same?

Making that decision provides much-needed focus on our day-to-day choices, which gives us a better sense of control in our lives and obliterates excuses. You're less likely to be disappointed if you consciously decide how to live and then live by those choices. No matter where you are in your journey to stay fit, keep at it. Remember who you are while sitting in that minivan. Stay true to that woman.

Multitasking Mania

"I don't know how she does it!" Maybe you think that about a mom you know, or perhaps people say that about you. Who knows how any of us manage to do everything we do. The fact is, sometimes we're afraid to stop and analyze our schedules. Sometimes this is because if we stop, we might not be able to start again. Who has time to think? Besides, thinking can evoke feelings, as in, "Doing this is a waste of my time," or "I don't *feel* like doing this." In other words, multitasking is a great tool *so long as you're multitasking those things that are priorities in your life.* Getting a grip on your priorities, however, actually requires you to think about what they are.

Obviously one of your priorities is fitness or you wouldn't be reading this book. You don't shirk your duties as a mother (or any of your other roles) in order to work out; that's why you're a champion multitasker. The happiest moms often include fitness in the process of mothering, a task you'll master by book's end. Still, we know finding enough time—any time for that matter—might be a daily struggle.

Energy Drain

Even when we're lucky enough to find the time to work out, sometimes the energy required is lost. This can be one of the unpleasant side effects of multitasking. Aside from reminding ourselves that there truly are only twenty-four hours in a day, we have to be realistic about what we can accomplish in our waking hours (because, yes, you do need sleep).

You need to eat right, too. This can be another challenge when your children's never-ending requests at mealtime rarely allow you to sit down at the table. Maintaining your energy might even require extra boosts, such as healthy snacks and supplements. We are in favor of legal stimulants, too. This book would not have been possible without copious amounts of coffee.

MOM 2 MOM

Keeping an exercise regimen gives me a feeling of control. Being a mom involves relinquishing control over almost all aspects of life—schedule, to-do list, personal needs—but when I make the effort to work out, I'm carving out some small piece of life that still feels like I run it, and it gives me energy.

—Karen, mom of two
San Jose, California

Guilt Trips

If we all believe fitness is a priority, why is a guilt-free workout so hard? Perhaps you've overcome *that* guilt but can't shake the feeling that you're not doing enough. No matter what we do or don't do, we usually end up feeling guilty for one reason or another. But the more confident we feel about our decisions the less likely we are to have any negative feelings associated with them.

The skill of "being present" is also extremely useful. Whatever you're doing—enjoy the moment. Stop fretting about other places you think you should be or other things you think you should be doing. (We're assuming here that you're not locked in the closet with a value-size bag of M&M's.) Wherever you are, whatever you're doing, be guilt-free—live in the here and now. Easier said than done. We know this is a lifelong pursuit, but we'll give you some concrete ideas on how to put this to work in your life as a fit mom.

There is always something that needs to be done, something that competes for my time. School always needs volunteers, and that is probably where I feel the most guilty; I have never made it to a PTA meeting, ever.

—Kami, mom of three
Yardley, Pennsylvania

Chaos

As moms, we really don't ever know exactly what to expect on a given day. Just when life begins to feel a bit routine, when we think we can start planning a little more—that is, take more time for ourselves—we are thrown a curveball and our workouts become out of reach. Sick kids, a science project ("It's due tomorrow, Mom!"), swimming lessons that run late, and canceled playdates are just a few of the things that might throw off your fitness regimen. Sometimes you might actually be in the midst of your workout when somebody—not just the kids—needs you and your fitness gets shortchanged again.

We're not talking about looking for excuses or an easy way to opt out of your workout. We're talking about being realistic. Sometimes a workout just isn't in the cards, and you have to give in. There was a mention about the world no longer revolving around you in the fine print when you became a parent, but in all the excitement, perhaps you didn't notice. Maybe over time you forgot. Maybe, just this once, just for today, you thought you found a loophole in the contract. As much as you feel like throwing a tantrum, resist the urge and embrace the chaos.

Forgetting What's Important

While we're busting hump to get to the gym—you know, to preserve our identity (OK, maybe the waistline, too)—we need not forget there are other good reasons to be there. Breaking a sweat reduces your risk of heart disease, as well as obesity and all the things that come with that—diabetes, hypertension, and stroke. Working out on a regular basis wards off osteoporosis, high cholesterol, and, ironically, fatigue. As you begin to commit more time to your fitness regimen, the benefits add up—well beyond becoming faster and stronger. And don't forget, you have to take care of yourself in order to best care for your children.

We've realized something else in our quest for fitness. Sweat dripping from your face is no longer considered unladylike. It now represents something wonderful—your inner strength. A good sweat reminds you of how far you've come, where you're going, and that you can survive this workout, this day, this year.

Sweaty gym clothes may be the first step in overcoming low self-esteem, depression, or just a plain old case of the blahs. We all have something to gain physically and mentally.

You're in Good Company

More women are turning to fitness than ever before. While these women all value physical activity, their mode of fitness varies. How a woman chooses to become fit is as unique as her sense of style. We won't provide any specific workouts in this book, because in order to make fitness part of your lifestyle it has to be something you're passionate about. There isn't a one-size-fits-all workout for that.

We have attempted to recognize the various types of moms and their different needs while writing this book. At our core, we all want the same thing: to be fit and stay sane in the process. With that we have culled five secrets for success and are sharing them here with you. But the following information shouldn't stay secret. Share your knowledge with your friends, your sisters, even your mother. It's never too late to be a Hot (Sweaty) Mama.

MOM 2 MOM

Children are constantly bombarded with unhealthy images, whether pictures of skeletal actresses or ads for fast food. I exercise so that they see it's one of the things we do to stay healthy and take care of our bodies.

—Kayris, mom of two
Baltimore, Maryland

I think there's nothing more beautiful than a strong, sweaty woman crossing the finish line in victory.

—Whitney, mom of three
Winter Springs, Florida

Secret Number One

YOU HAVE TO
TRAIN YOUR BRAIN
BEFORE YOU CAN
TRAIN YOUR BODY

one

SIDELINE PRECONCEPTIONS AND SET PRIORITIES

If being a mom is hard work and being fit is hard work, logic tells us that being a fit mom is the mother of all challenges.

You may have been up for the challenge since sperm met egg. Or maybe you can't fathom adding anything else to your already hectic life; it's like grabbing *just one more* grocery bag on your way into the house. Dare you risk everything falling apart?

Being fit before having children doesn't necessarily give you the upper hand. Whether you were on bed rest, lifting no more than the remote control, or ran on the day you gave birth is irrelevant. Maybe someone else carried your baby. It doesn't matter. Nine months come and go, but raising children takes eighteen years or more. Any mom who wants to get the sweat out of her system is left with the same dilemma: How do I get my workout in *now*?

Often the perceived solution is based on preconceptions and misconceptions we acquired before having children. For instance: Work out when the baby naps. In a perfect world you would start that exercise DVD and turn on the baby monitor. In the imperfect world, where most of us live, ten minutes later the monitor is lighting up and you haven't even hit your stride.

There's also that preconception about how *your* children will never watch television. Never say never. The notion of a "captive audience" makes a lot of sense when you realize a Disney video is your ticket to thirty minutes of yoga or those free-weight exercises you dog-eared in your favorite fitness magazine.

Now that you're a mother—with nothing left to imagination—you know there will be days when workouts will need to be squeezed in between feedings, when you may get interrupted during kickboxing class to change a poopy diaper, when yoga will be preempted by Little League, and even times, yes, when you simply will be too exhausted to move another step.

These are universal dilemmas for fit moms everywhere. Some days these issues are little hiccups in our day; other times we feel like the groove is gone and lost forever. But you can be committed to both motherhood and fitness. Sure, the more you want to work out, the more planning it will take on the front end. That planning requires you to stay true to yourself and what is important to you.

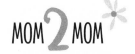

Lose Misconceptions with the Baby Fat

Right after that second line appeared on your home pregnancy test you probably began daydreaming about picture-perfect moments: You and your baby staring lovingly into each other's eyes, first smiles, little fingers, pacifiers, books, and lullabies. In your fairy-tale version of parenting, your baby slept through the night, ate on a regular schedule, and never projectile vomited onto your favorite shirt. You were impressed by how quickly you got your prebaby body back. As your baby grew, she potty-trained easily, could read before starting kindergarten, and suggested the family participate in volunteer activities every holiday. She didn't have an uncontrollable temper tantrum when it was time to leave the park, she didn't color her nose with a blue Sharpie right before a scheduled portrait, and she didn't pretend you weren't her mom as she got older. How's that for ignorance?

If not for these preconceptions, adapting to the realities of motherhood might not be so hard. We make it harder than it needs to be because we let the media get to us with all those celebrity cover girls in bikinis two weeks postpartum. We allow our vision of the perfect, fit mother to rule our psyche. We fail to acknowledge misconceptions as false, unattainable, and detrimental.

We've all looked at another mother and thought, "I should be like her." The reality, however, is that the "ideal mom" probably feels like she's coming apart at the seams, too. So when you see another mom working out, be secure in the fact that her circumstances are different from yours and she probably has "those moments," too.

When it comes to renewing or developing your identity as a fit mom—for your sanity, your health, and your happiness—you have to lose the preconceptions and misconceptions about motherhood you're hanging on to and determine what is realistic for you to accomplish *now*.

Take Inventory

It's time to take inventory of your life. What is it you value most? How do these values translate into priorities? How do these priorities guide your day? Write them down. Commit them to memory. Make them part of your subconscious. Post them where you can see them: your bathroom mirror, the refrigerator door, the dashboard of the car. Then in the midst of a busy day, you'll have a frequent reminder of what's really important when "outside influences" make you second-guess your priorities or try to add to your list.

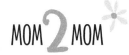

My biggest battle is my inner exercise addict versus my inner neat freak. I really need an orderly environment, and when I work out in lieu of housecleaning I just feel icky. Not guilty, exactly; just icky.

—Susan, mom of three
Harrisburg, Pennsylvania

Try this for starters. Grab a notebook and keep a log of your activities for one full (typical) day. There's no need for elaborate entries; just jot down a list of where and how you're spending your time throughout the day. Then, at the end of the day, categorize your actions (for example, career, mommy chores, family time, philanthropy, personal enrichment, fitness, and so on). Next, highlight or circle those categories that you consider values in your life. Are you spending your time in your most valuable areas? Whether you like it or not, where you allot the most time translates into your actual priorities. So, are your *perceived priorities* in line with your *actual priorities*? An exercise like this helps us see the truth about how we spend our time. See "Fit Mom Inventory and Examples" in the appendix for help.

Protect Your Priorities as Ruthlessly as Your Children

As you work at reconciling your actual priorities with your perceived priorities, make sure you are clear about what's important to you. It goes without saying that one of your greatest priorities may, at this very moment, be attached to your leg screaming, "Mama! Mama!" Much like your own children, your highest priorities in life should be easy to identify (not necessarily clinging and screaming for your attention, though). They don't always have physical characteristics (dimpled chins or sparkling eyes), but our priorities need to be nurtured just like our kids.

Most of us consider family, friends, faith, philanthropic pursuits, or career high on the priority list. Because you're reading this book, we're certain that health and fitness rank up there, too. Priorities give our life shape, meaning, and—this is important—structure. It's your own unique mix of priorities that makes you who you are, but only if you have the courage to live by them.

This is more than time management, because if you don't know who you want to be, then you don't know how to spend your time. Once you are clear about your priorities it's easier to make decisions—say yes, say no—in order to spend your precious time honoring that person—those ideals, those goals, those dreams.

It all sounds good in theory: Do what is most important to you. But there's this ugly little demon called "mother guilt" that some of us carry around like an ankle weight on our hearts. It can drag us down even when we know we're doing what is right for our families and ourselves.

MOM 2 MOM

There have been times my kids have missed a playgroup because I have a commitment to myself and the gym. I do, however, make it up afterward with a trip to the park or a group bike ride.

—Melissa, mom of three
Turlock, California

Your child screaming as you drop him off at the gym's day care so that you can attend to another one of your priorities is such an example. You feel that temptation to snatch him back, drive him home, and hold him tightly until he graduates from college. Don't be silly. Mother guilt truly has no place in your life if you've established your priorities correctly. And like those of us with multiple children know, you can have more than one priority in your life just as you can love and nurture more than one child. What's a little sibling rivalry?

True contentment—that happy place where the pendulum rests—is found when we realistically dedicate the right amount of time to our various priorities. Just for emphasis: We said the *right* amount of time. That, friend, is the difference between frustration and contentment, and contentment and *guilt*. Not enough time spent on a priority leads to frustration. Too much time in one area creates guilt.

Sometimes the problem isn't a life without direction or finding the right balance among our priorities so much as the dreaded "yes" disease. Even when we're very clear about our priorities we often get sucked into spending our time in ways that don't serve our priorities so well. Why? Who knows? It sounded like a good idea at the time? We want people to like us? We're flattered they asked or think us competent to handle the request? Keep saying yes and there goes your fitness, date night with your husband, even that ten minutes you need alone in the bathroom.

Have you ever noticed that when you're busy tending to your priorities—allocating the right amount of time to each—being busy feels good? In fact, you marvel at your efficiency and lack of stress while you are getting so much accomplished.

And then there's harried busy, the "Why am I doing this?" busy. The kind of busy that causes headaches, sleepless nights, illness, injury, and (this is a big one) *unhappiness*. Are you doing a lot of complaining? And worse, are you critical of people who *are* happy? Sure signs you're two-timing your priorities.

I struggle with mother guilt on a daily basis. Seems like no matter what I do for myself, there is always a little voice in my head (sometimes in the room) telling me I should be doing something else—something for someone else. It's hard work ignoring mother guilt, but, the truth is, I'm a much better mom when I do. Ultimately, I break down both physically and mentally when I forget to make myself a priority in my life. And that just leaves even less of me to share with my family.

—Laurie

MOM 2 MOM

Because I work out early in the morning I say no to so many evening things and I still often feel guilty missing parties, dinners, hanging out, and so on. I've earned myself a reputation. Hopefully for more than being an early bird, though.

—Misha, mom of two
Bellingham, Washington

Perhaps the most important time-management tool we have is the ability to listen—and respond—to our bodies. So steer clear of those unpleasant physical symptoms by staying true to yourself. Set boundaries around your priorities and make them impenetrable to "other things" that may provide only fleeting contentment and hollow feelings of accomplishment.

As mothers we've had a lot of practice saying "no" to our kids. Now, when you need to, make sure you can say it to other people (and sometimes yourself).

Don't Let Temporary Imbalances Throw Off Your High-Wire Act

Sometimes life throws us off balance, and to avoid hitting the ground below we have to say "no" to something that is a high priority. Life changes—another baby comes along, you move your family across the country, a parent becomes ill—any of these things can take up greater space in your life, demanding you scale back somewhere. If you're already spending time the way you want to, this can be painful, even downright scary, especially if you have to trim back on things that define you. This is certainly harder than saying no to a low-priority activity, but if you say no consciously—on purpose, with forethought and intent—then you keep some control over your life. The ability to say "no" is your safety net.

Deciding to put something on hold isn't "giving up." You're not pushing the "eject" button, just hitting "pause." You can come back when you're ready. The decision allows you to feel empowered, versus feeling like you're drowning in "too much to do" or—even worse—feeling like a failure if you physically, mentally, and emotionally can't keep up with it all.

Sometimes it's not the big, life-changing events that catch us off guard, but smaller, short-term upheavals. Whenever possible, try to anticipate and adjust to these short-term

> My life was "temporarily imbalanced" the summer I had three children under age two. I made the decision to take a sabbatical from freelance writing as well as scale back on running and triathlon training. I was sorely lacking confidence as a mother and I knew the remedy was to strengthen my mothering skills. Whenever I felt the need to breathe in a paper bag, I quickly reminded myself that I was in charge of this decision and would eventually return to my roles as writer and athlete. When I did, my life was better equipped to encompass all I ask of it.
>
> —Kara

imbalances—those days or months that are more hectic than others. Perhaps Thursdays are particularly crazy. Maybe it's the start of the school year, the holidays, tax season. Prepare yourself by planning ahead how you will scale back or otherwise make it work. Again, being a step ahead ensures that you (or your fitness routine) don't become the victim of being too busy. And if you do cut back, you don't have to feel angry or cheated. It didn't *happen* to you. You made that choice (and you know it's temporary).

The good news is that your fitness doesn't have to fall away from your universe if life gets too extreme. Sometimes it only requires *lowering* your expectations. No, that doesn't make you a quitter. It just means acknowledging the validity of what you can realistically accomplish; for example, a short walk to the park is worthy of logging in your exercise journal. (And we'll convince you of that later.)

Speaking of convincing, have we persuaded you that fitness should be a priority? If you're not quite there yet, read on. Perhaps you are still waffling about your decision to get fit. In the next chapter, we'll help you make that commitment for good.

MOM **2** MOM

When I am not working full-time, volunteering at the school, driving a kid somewhere, or hitting Target at 10 p.m., something or someone is always asking for my time. Workouts are a treat for me.

—Lara, mom of two
Richfield, Minnesota

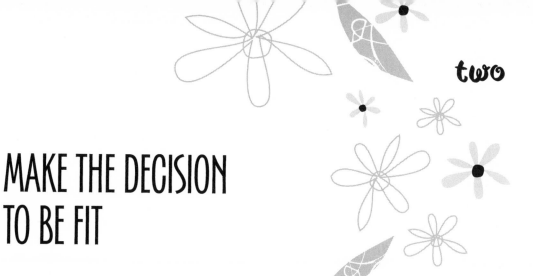

two

MAKE THE DECISION TO BE FIT

If you're like a lot of moms out there, you've probably made a number of starts and stops in the pursuit of fitness. No matter how hard you've tried, exercise never became a habit. Maybe it wasn't fun. Perhaps it actually hurt—and not in the "good pain" sort of way. It might have even been a bit lonely, too.

Nodding your head? You may not be active right now, but you want to be, right? And you believe in the merits of exercise, too, don't you? Yet fitness just isn't a functioning part of your life yet. What does it take to make your intentions a reality?

It all boils down to motivation. Exercise probably won't become part of your lifestyle if you rely on a single motivator—for example, weight loss, because your friend talked you into joining the gym, or because "it's the right thing to do." Sure, any one of these reasons will do a great job of getting you started down the path of fitness, but it may not provide enough force to sustain a fit *life*. A list of good reasons, though—including those mentioned above—can create synergy for your motivation. On some days that "one good reason to exercise" might fail you, but with five others on the list, how can you refuse?

Over time, those things that motivated you to start exercising (like the extra weight, the gym membership, the doctor's orders) become less important. They peel away to reveal a new motivation—one that comes from within and has nothing to do with what size jeans you wear or even your cholesterol level.

Why Do You Exercise?

Tops on the list for most moms in our survey are stress reduction, needing "me time," weight management, social time with workout partners, and modeling healthy behavior to the kids. A few other reasons fall outside the box. Any of these reasons sound familiar or seem like a good reason to work up a sweat yourself?

- It makes me remember that while I am a mom (taxi driver, cook, nurse, maid, and so on), I am still a real person as well!
- I want my kids, especially my daughter, to see a mom who is fit and not obsessing about her body.
- To feel happy!
- I was never the athletic kid or the skinny kid (I am still not skinny), but the pride I have in my newfound strength keeps me going.
- It allows me time to pray and time to appreciate being outside.
- To stay sexy after forty!
- When I exercise I am less likely to sink into self-pity.
- I am a type 1 diabetic, and I don't want anyone to think this disease can stop me from living the life I want to lead.
- I have boys. I don't want to be a boring couch potato mom who can't be active with them.
- I like demonstrating to my daughters that Mom—although "really old" at fifty—can still get around.
- It helps me get my head on straight. I feel better organized after I am done.
- I have a spectacularly unhealthy mom myself, and I'd really like to enjoy old age in ways that are not possible for her.
- I call it reality reduction time—and it's all mine!
- To keep me centered and spiritually present.
- I am a better mom when I can beat out my frustrations on a spin bike or weights rather than take it out on the kids!
- So that when I am eighty plus, I can bend over and pick up my grandkids!
- I feel more alive when I sweat.

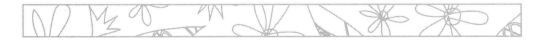

Make Exercise a Habit

Motivation is essential in forming a habit. It isn't, however, the only thing required. No, it takes a good acronym for that. Turn fitness from a dreaded task into a HABIT with these criteria:

Happy inducing
Authentic activity
Better off after than before
Integrates easily into life
Time valued

Happy Inducing

There is a T-shirt out there that says, "Running is my Prozac." We can laugh at it in a dismissive way, yet plenty of research and personal anecdotes (and our firsthand experience) supports the fact that exercise is a mood enhancer. Elevate your heart rate, elevate your endorphins—they're those fun-loving neurotransmitters that travel around your brain looking for a party.

> Like any notable first (ahem), I remember the first run that resulted in an endorphin high. That's when I realized I had to run longer than my usual two miles for the party to start.
>
> —Kara

Fitness advocates know this about regular exercise; they've experienced it time and time again. In fact, the body becomes accustomed to those endorphins and with too many sedentary days it will long for a mood-lifting workout. It's as if your brain is saying, "Where's the party?" So we can laugh in the same dismissive way when someone says, "I'm addicted to exercise," because in some respects it's true. Miss more than a few days, and you're sure to notice.

Still, if you never experienced these little cephalic parties, how can you know what you're missing or believe in the benefit? The kind of "happy inducing" most women are after is the kind they can see in the mirror: a smaller waistline and thinner thighs. Even then, in our instant-gratification society, good old exercise can't deliver fast enough—certainly not like cosmetic surgery can. Women who undergo surgical enhancements often list the same reasons why other women exercise: "to make me happy" or "to feel better about myself."

Granted, liposuction and tummy tucks can work miracles on the physical self. Who wouldn't be happy to wake up and find excess flab gone? But being fit via slow and steady exercise can transform the body in ways plastic surgery can't, namely a healthier heart (which betters your odds of seeing your children grow up), improved stamina (to keep up with the rigors of motherhood), and increased muscle mass (giving you confidence when wearing that little black dress). There's also a mental transformation that goes along with regular exercise and—this is important—goal setting. Now we're talking about more than improved mood. Along with your exercise you get sides of self-confidence, resolve, persistence, and power. None of that is available post-op.

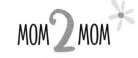

We're certain that the end result of a good workout is happy inducing, but to get to those ends you need happy-inducing means.

Depression

For many women, happy-inducing effects are the main reason they exercise: to get up, get moving, and feel the problems of the day ooze out of their pores right along with the sweat. For some women, the clinical effect is even greater: Exercise treats or prevents their depression.

- Since I went off my antidepressants, I feel very attached to exercise to ward off evil bouts with depression and anxious thoughts. I am happier as a mom, and think I have a happier child and husband because of it.
- I'd have to double up on the Zoloft if I didn't have my therapy time with my running buddy.
- Exercise is my antidepressant. It's my sanity. My brain is chemically dependent on it. Without it, watch out.
- I had a physician's assistant order me to start running when I asked her for antidepressants. She told me my depression was situational and pills wouldn't change that. Running has helped me tremendously even though I hated it at first. Now I love it.
- Exercise is the best antidepression medication I could ever ask for. And at the best price too!

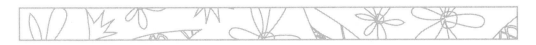

Authentic Activity

The staple of staying motivated and true to a fit lifestyle is knowing what mode of movement feels authentic—the kind of exercise that correlates with your personality and becomes an expression of yourself. That's typically not a one-size-fits-all workout plan. You're going to have to dig a little deeper.

Finding your authentic activity (and, hey, let's be positive and say "activities") can be hit or miss. First you need to experiment, explore fitness options, and find something that moves you in more ways than one.

This means you'll have to try new things. It means you may put yourself in situations where you might feel intimidated, even silly. (We tried a hip-hop dance class once, so we speak from experience.) What activities did you enjoy as a kid? Chances are if you enjoyed it then, you'll enjoy it now. If you're a member of a health club, set out to try one new fitness class a week. Don't limit yourself to the indoors though.

My problem is I have experimented so much I now have FADD (fitness attention deficit disorder). There are so many activities I love to do, want to improve at, or still want to try.

—Kara

Just as you tend to buy food according to what's in season, so it is with exercise. If you live in winter climes, try cross-country skiing or snowshoeing. Think local, too. Live near the ocean? How about surfing? Is a lake nearby? Take a lesson in kayaking or canoeing. In fact, your authentic activities are easier to discover if you pursue a fitness journey, a mission to find yourself in activity. And this journey is never over, by the way. Never be afraid to try new things.

While you're out there experimenting, be careful not to dismiss anything too quickly. Remember when you were introducing new foods to your baby? The rule is to expose your child to a new food four or five times before assuming they're spitting it back at you for good reason. It takes that many tries to turn on those taste buds. You might need as many tries to give something new a chance, too.

Eventually your activities of choice will become who you are, another layer in your identity. When you fill out that line on paperwork that asks for "favorite activities or hobbies," you write down the things that you love. Whatever you choose to do for exercise you must love in the same way.

Better Off After Than Before

Even those of us who have discovered our authentic activity sometimes still need a shove to get out the door. That "shove" is often just knowing that we'll feel better after our workout is over—both physically and mentally, but also in the sense of empowerment that comes from following through. Anytime you can check something off your "list," you feel more capable.

Still, there certainly are a lot of steps to get through before coming out the other side happy you made the effort. Take, for instance, running—an activity we both love to do. But to do it, we often have to get up before the sun. Where we live, most morning runs require "suiting up" in several layers. We like to push ourselves, so there's usually some discomfort involved in the process, and sometimes some residual soreness, too. So, how do you express to someone who doesn't exercise that it's all good? That running isn't a burden, but a luxury (especially since becoming a mom you rarely get time alone). That having that workout behind us puts a positive spin on the rest of our day?

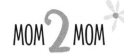

MOM 2 MOM

It's a tough sell, for sure, or everyone would be exercising. Like the endorphin high, it's not a tangible benefit—you can experience it only after you've put in the hard work. But the outcome—that benefit—is definitely *worth* the hard work.

Have you ever said this to yourself after a workout: "Geez . . . I sure wish I hadn't exercised"?

Integrates Easily into Life

You might really love to downhill ski. But you live in Kansas City. You might really love field hockey. But as a working mom, you have time only to suit up before you run out of "me time." This doesn't mean you can no longer ski or play field hockey, but those activities won't be the main part of your fitness routine.

To make exercise a part of your life you not only have to love it, but it has to love you back. It should fit into your life like another family member or a beloved pet. Would you consider bringing a long-haired cat into your home if your spouse was allergic to cats? Would a black lab pup be a good choice for a busy family without a yard? If you're choosing the next family pet, you'd do your homework and find an animal well suited to your personality, your schedule, and your lifestyle. Finding the right mode of exercise is similar. It can be neither too burdensome to pursue nor too time consuming. It has to be a good fit with everything else you're already doing.

Time Valued

As you know, time is precious, and it's only natural for you to spend it in those areas that bring you the most bang for your buck. Once you have found your authentic activities that are well suited to your lifestyle and have reaped the benefits of regular exercise, those activities will begin to rank higher in your day. You will actually value the time you spend exercising—not just positive side effects like losing weight or spending time with friends—but the very *act* of exercising. You might start thinking, "I *get* to do this!"

You'll notice some wonderful changes in your behavior, too. You'll spend less time in front of the television, less time shopping, and less time obsessing over what junk food might be hidden in the back of your cupboards. Once you weed out those activities, you'll start to wonder what you did with all your time before exercise became one of your must-do activities.

> After my first daughter was born, I was excited to get rid of pants with elastic waistbands and oversized shirts. I couldn't wait to put on "normal" clothes and was shocked when nothing fit me. I thought for sure I could squeeze into my loose jeans for the trip home from the hospital; naively, I even packed them in my hospital bag. Daily attempts at stuffing myself in my prebaby clothes got me out walking, then running, as soon as possible. What began as an effort to lose the baby weight turned into precious alone time spent meditating and centering on my new life. Eight years later, I still use fitness to calm my mind.
>
> —Laurie

Empowered by Exercise

Once you've succeeded at maintaining a regular exercise schedule (check the appendix for the "Twenty-Eight-Day Fitness Challenge" if you need more help making exercise a habit) two benefits will follow that will likely close the deal. One is the physical benefit—you'll literally experience progress, whether that's weight loss, improved muscle tone, or lower cholesterol. The second is a gain in performance. You'll notice that you can go faster on the treadmill, you last longer in step class, or you can move deeper into a yoga pose. Those physical benefits are often enough to feed the motivation. Feeling good begets feeling good. In this way, exercise is somewhat addicting above and beyond the endorphin high.

Yes, some people can take it to extremes and abuse exercise, much like an eating disorder, but that's not what we're talking about. We're talking about exercise now as a habit—like your morning caffeine, the order in which you load the dishwasher, the way you like to drive to work, or your bedtime routine.

The reason exercise becomes habit-forming is because it provides you with a sense of power over your life: You can control what you do with your day and take time to do something that makes you feel good. It literally makes you feel strong and powerful. Exercise is a bridge between mind and body, and it empowers them both. Once you've been exposed to that power (like the endorphins) it's hard to give up. This positive force is self-perpetuating. Now fitness is more than a habit; it's a lifestyle.

Fitness as a Lifestyle

Fitness is a metamorphosis from a desire to be healthy to a commitment to an active life—to keeping your body at a higher level of conditioning. Where once you socialized at the coffee shop after dropping the kids off at preschool, you now make a beeline to the gym. Where once you took a power lunch at work, now you take a power walk. But you're hardly alone in your pursuits. Those who call you friend are likely to mix and mingle on the move.

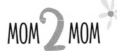

MOM 2 MOM

I lost a significant amount of weight and when my pants kept falling down during yoga class and exposing my squishy mommy tummy—now with extra flaps of skin!—I realized my time to buy smaller workout clothes had come. I picked out running capris, a wicking tee, extra athletic socks, and a pack of small bath towels for my gym bag. When I stacked the merchandise on the counter and saw what I was buying, I almost started to cry. Until then, I hadn't noticed that I went to the sporting goods store to buy clothes I *needed*, not just clothes that I aspire to need. Because I am a swimmer, I am a runner, I am a person who takes new exercise classes just for the heck of it; I am a person who never misses a workout. I had become that person.

—Erin, mom of four
Minneapolis, Minnesota

Women who embrace a fit lifestyle invest in the essentials. Finding a good jog bra is just as important as buying that top-of-the-line baby jogger or bike trailer. Who cares if the minivan doesn't fit in the garage? What's most important is that workouts fit into your day. Having workout clothes at the ready and being able to easily switch gears if the opportunity to work out presents itself is part of the fit-lifestyle mentality.

We can try to convince you in all kinds of ways to become fit. We'll keep telling you how important it is to include exercise in your life, but in the end it boils down to making the decision. Stop hemming and hawing; stop analyzing. Start doing. All of life's big decisions are like that, too: marriage, children, career—you just have to make the decision. Are you in or are you out?

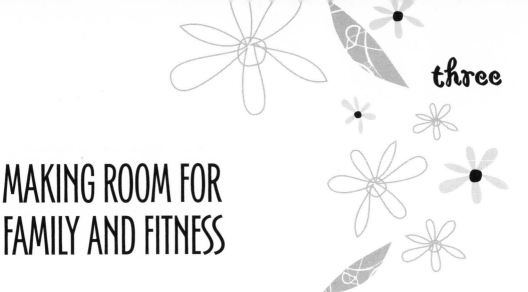

three

MAKING ROOM FOR FAMILY AND FITNESS

It doesn't matter whether you're adding a family to your active lifestyle or trying to add an active lifestyle into family life; either way you want to do more. We've all had those moments when we stopped to wonder: Will another car seat fit in the second row? Can we squeeze one more box of frozen waffles into the freezer? Is it possible to stuff one more towel in the washing machine? And isn't the answer always *yes*? Don't you make it work?

While fitting exercise into your life is more of a mental riddle, as we've solved in the first two chapters, sometimes it takes a little mental muscle to physically squeeze and stuff those workouts into our day.

If you aren't already ultraorganized and superefficient (we know that woman exists and we'd love to make her our new best friend), adopting some or all of these ways to expand your day can give your life more room to wedge in a workout. Sometimes you can use the extra space for other things: more time to spend helping on homework, cuddle time with your spouse, cooking meals. Ideally, over the course of a week, you might feel a sense of . . . what is that holy grail for busy moms? Oh yes, *balance*.

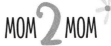

MOM **2** MOM

I am a single mom, and exercise is the fuel that keeps my life in order. Though it adds another demand for time, it makes me more productive throughout the rest of the day.

—Debra, mom of one
Atlanta, Georgia

Balance is a wily cat. Sometimes he sits in our lap, content to stay. Other times he'll dash off and hide for days. But balance returns. Now, what can we do to attract balance? How do we get balance to come around more often? Get balance to stay with us longer?

Catnip.

The kind of catnip that attracts balance to our life is the same brand of action we take to expand our day. Our strategy starts with a schedule; our tactics involve triaging our to-do list. We can make enough room in our life for family *and* fitness.

Mental Housekeeping

Let's be clear. Managing our life doesn't necessarily mean creating order. Step into our homes unannounced and you'll likely be introduced to a little chaos. Perhaps you're familiar with the antics of the quasi-potty-trained toddler. Dogs provide the first line of defense for cleaning the kitchen floor. Artwork hangs from every wall by six inches of tangled Scotch tape. Shoes litter the entryway, oftentimes without their mates. Dirty clothes land anywhere but *in* the laundry basket. And before the dinner dishes are even washed, there are kids screaming for snacks and drinks.

No matter how much we try to keep things orderly, life doesn't lend itself to order. It's as if with the simple act of breathing, clutter returns. (Fitness is kind of like that, too. You never reach a point when you can stop eating healthfully, or when you no longer need to exercise because you've reached maximum fitness.) The laundry will never be "done." The floor will need to be swept again, eventually. And, oh, how we love those dishwashers, if only they could empty themselves.

How do we keep it all together? It's the *mental* housekeeping that keeps an active mom's life more orderly. Part of the fit-mom learning curve involves figuring out what you can do to help yourself function as efficiently as possible. That starts with a schedule.

The word *schedule* gets a bad rap. Even though we know the intent of a schedule is to

> I schedule three or four early morning workouts during the week. The rest of my week is more flexible; I plan workouts the night before or sometimes that same day. For me, it's the perfect mix of planning and spontaneity. Usually one workout gets bumped, which leaves me with six days of exercise each week. I'm happy with that.
>
> —Laurie

help bring order to our lives, free spirits of the world tend toward spontaneity and freedom. If the idea of a schedule sounds too rigid to you, you may be missing out on many of life's big and small accomplishments.

A schedule doesn't have to be rigid. A schedule can be nothing more than our intentions for the day, the week, the month. A schedule allows us to be proactive so we can integrate our own plan with the activities of our children, partners, and other obligations.

In reality, much of our time spent as moms is reactive: baby poops, you change the diaper; child runs through house with muddy shoes, you call your neighbor to borrow her steam cleaner; boss asks you to work late, you scramble to engage the emergency car pool. Some situations we simply can't anticipate, nor would we want to write them on our calendar. But by anticipating any lulls and putting a plan in place to exercise, we *can* be proactive and take control. Carpe diem!

> I've been the mom who forgets to bring snacks to school. I have a day planner and I write things down, but, yes, sometimes I forget to look at my calendar. If an additional responsibility comes up, I better write it down in more than one place: For me that's the "family bulletin board" in the kitchen.
>
> —Kara

A schedule, in the life of a mom, is more like a battle plan. It outlines how you want to engage, but you have to be able to react to enemy forces; you have to know when to attack or to retreat, when to fall back on Plan B or develop Plan C on the fly.

Our mission is to turn intention into reality as often as possible.

Start with what you know. What happens on a daily, weekly, or monthly basis that is predictable? That's the foundation for your schedule; that's the structure you have to build on.

A system to track your obligations provides a means to get them out of your brain (where they are taking up valuable memory—you know you need more) and onto a calendar, whiteboard, notepad, smart phone, or the palm of your hand. Now your brain has space to handle other matters (perhaps remembering to bring snacks or to pick up toilet paper on the way home from work). Whatever system works for you, it's a road map for your days and weeks ahead. Having a system for tracking your schedule prevents you from being a flake. Really. Your kids do not want you to be the mom who forgets the snacks.

Next, scrutinize your schedule. How much real time is left? What other things happen that are so entrenched in your daily routine that you fail to count them because you hardly think about them—such as letting out the dog, who needs just the right location and conditions to pee? What about the tasks that you think should take no time at all, but in a children's world drag on—such as getting into the car? What about the trivial mommy tasks that, while you can do them with your eyes closed, still take time, such as restocking the diaper bag? Even minutiae takes real time. We might forget that our day is full with what is already happening.

Can you simplify your schedule? Are you unintentionally making life more complex than it needs to be? A major step in simplifying life happens when you eliminate what's unnecessary. The less you have the less you have to deal with. If you cancel all those catalogs you never look at, you save yourself the step of throwing them away (not to mention a tree or two). If you pay your bills online, you save yourself the step of opening mail (and another tree). Make yourself a master grocery list and don't throw it away. Consider all the products you use in a day. Are they all necessary? Could you live without applying one, two, or three of them? The cumulative minutes you save could add up.

Once you have a realistic picture of your schedule, pay close attention. What works well in your schedule and what doesn't? Can you conquer some of that pithy stuff a day ahead or put it off until tomorrow? Often, it's prep work the day before that can make the next day run more smoothly: making lunch the night before, packing backpacks and gym bags, then loading the car all before you hit the hay. Know which mornings lend themselves to pancakes and which ones are better suited for granola bars.

If you ever have those fleeting sensations that being a mom is easy, then something clicked in your day in a major way. Figure out what just happened and repeat it as often as possible. When you discover something that works well, adopt it as an official part

MOM 2 MOM

I get up at 4:30 a.m. three days a week, nurse my five-month-old while pumping the other breast, change her, dress her, and put her back down to sleep, all so I can get out early and have her be ready for my husband to wake up and take to the sitter on the days I work.

—Amanda, mom of two
McCallsburg, Iowa

I signed up for karate with my son. I'd rather work out than sit on my rump in a waiting room.

—Jocelyn, mom of three
Maple Grove, Minnesota

of your schedule. The idea is to create systems to streamline and make your life feel easier. When something is easier it can leave us energy for other things, like a workout.

Pay attention to the places in your day where you can squeeze something else in. Maybe it's signing your kids up for a swim lesson at a time when you can work in a few laps yourself. Maybe a playdate goes so well—as in, the kids all play while you finish an exercise video—that you make it a weekly occurrence (don't ask how having more kids in the house can allow you a gulp of sanity, but we know it can).

Part of the fit-mom learning curve involves figuring out what you can do to help yourself function as efficiently as possible. Mental housekeeping clears out space and cleans up your schedule; you have to control the clutter in your mind to prevent clutter from controlling your life.

File To-Do List Bankruptcy

Your schedule is an effective road map as long as you entrust yourself only to those appointments and actions you're actually committed to (work and school schedule, doctor's appointments, lessons, and so on). Otherwise, if everything is equally compelling, then what's really important? This shapes your obligations into something more manageable. And since your schedule is aligned with your personal priorities, exercise should be on your calendar most days of the week. It's on there, right?

As for that ever-growing, never-shrinking to-do list you started months ago? Throw it out. Filing to-do list bankruptcy absolves you of the long list of to-dos that might leave you feeling like that proverbial deer in the headlights, unable to get anything done because you can't figure out where to start. No, you'll never actually be absolved of your daily "debts," but filing to-do list bankruptcy gives you the opportunity to let go of unrealistic expectations.

So what about all those other things that you need to get to . . . eventually?

Have you had to take your child to the emergency room yet? (No? Your time will come.) Did you notice that patients emitting vomit or blood get seen right away? You can triage what needs to get done in your day in a similar fashion. On your list of actions, what might cause excessive bleeding or cause you to vomit if you don't get to it? Figuratively speaking, of course, but we're sure there are instances where it feels literal. What we're saying here is, focus on those things, and only those things, that must get done today.

This is an awesome excuse to hit the snooze button. While you're lying awake (albeit barely) but not quite ready to heave your body out of bed, call a meeting with yourself. "What *must* get done? What do I *want* to get done?"

You can triage while breast-feeding a baby at 4 a.m., on a morning run, while taking a shower, waiting for the coffee to brew, sitting in the carpool line (you get the drift). Just ask yourself, "What do I need to do *today*?"

Remember to be realistic. Limit your obligations. Three to five should be the max. You don't want your mind to end up like an overcrowded emergency room: You have only one day to tend to your "patients."

What's first? Allow us to continue with our blood/vomit analogy. It's gross, but you've seen it all before.

The blood represents those obligations that are already on your calendar. And the vomit, that's the emotions that direct your day by what you feel like doing. Sometimes we don't feel like going for a run if we have a sick child; sometimes the anxiety of a work deadline makes us feel like working late instead of heading to the gym. Likewise, a stressful week can give your workouts a sense of urgency, or anxiety about an upcoming 5K run can turn your primary attention toward training. Feelings are an important consideration when structuring your day. How you feel can determine the pecking order for your actions. Remember to take care of the blood first, but pay attention to that weak stomach or you'll be down for the count.

By mentally laying out your must-do tasks early in your day you will know when, or if, you'll get your workout in that day, and you won't be stressed trying to cram it in. If you make the decision that exercise won't be on the agenda, you won't be hard on yourself, because *you* made that decision to go without.

It wasn't until we wrote this chapter that I started employing this first-order-of-the-day task (you know, to walk the talk). Thing is, spending a few minutes in the morning to anticipate the day ahead and come up with a reasonable action plan really works for me, more than keeping a calendar or an ongoing list. If I can only focus on one day I don't feel overwhelmed and, to a certain extent, feel like I can be more "present." When I don't do this I feel like the Tasmanian devil, whirling around from one thing to the next, most often keeping busy being busy, but not accomplishing anything.

—Kara

Tomorrow you may choose to do something different under the same circumstances, or you may realize you can't do it alone.

Buy, Barter, or Beg

Sometimes there are things that never seem to get done despite our best efforts. Can't fathom another minute more of lost sleep? Have a big deadline looming at work? Can't go without another workout? It's time to enlist a little help: Clear chunks in your schedule by hiring a housekeeper, lawn boy, or handyman; use a personal assistant service; buy prepared meals and shop online.

Got the purse strings tied a little too tight for this? If you can afford it but can't get past spending the money on "frivolous expenditures," consider this: If you had to buy your workout, what would you pay? Invest in your sanity.

If you can't afford it, figure out how you can negotiate these services without breaking the bank. Pay the kid next door to mow the lawn, or ask the babysitter to run an errand or vacuum for you. Pick one day a month to make some meals ahead of time and stock your freezer. Maybe you don't like the way your husband folds clothes. Well, let it go and let him fold, and get back an hour in your week for something *important*. Maybe all it takes is developing a good chore list for the rest of the family. Shirking your duties? Absolutely not. You're teaching your children responsibility.

Another economical way to "get it all done" is to barter services. What are you good at? More precisely, what are you good at that you enjoy enough to do for someone else? The ideal situation, of course, is to relegate what you don't enjoy to someone else in trade. Let's say you hate to cook but you love organizing closets. Find that utterly disorganized gourmet friend. While she prepares a meal for you, tackle her closet.

You likely already barter your services. We barter when we share a car pool or swap kids for playdates. Just expand that thinking. I'll fold your laundry if you'll apply your green thumb to my flower bed. I'll walk your dog if you'll pick up my dry cleaning. I'll wash your car if you iron a few shirts for me. You get the idea.

There's one behavior all women need to master: asking for help.

Cyclists like to say there are two types of cyclists: those who have fallen off their bike and those who will. In some ways, life is a little like that, too. There are those who reach a point where they realize they need to ask for and accept the generosity of others, and those who aren't yet comfortable accepting help from others but are destined to get there.

Everyone has their "enough" point. For Laurie it was after struggling too long with postpartum depression. For Kara, it happened when she moved to a new state just before giving birth to twins. In both cases people reached out but for the first time in our lives we didn't deflect the help. Funny thing is, we weren't ashamed. Getting help feels good (it feels even better to the helper), so there's no reason to avoid this win-win situation.

Once you've accepted help it's easier to ask for it. Asking for help doesn't make you a wimpy woman. On the contrary, it's liberating. You're not asking for a crutch; you're asking for a boost—a little lift. If asking for the help you need gets you through your day, a difficult week, or a life crisis, then you've succeeded. The best way to show your gratitude for the help is to pay it forward. What mother in your neighborhood could use a little lift?

Just as time and experience allow us to become more comfortable as mothers, finding your way as a fit mom is similar. At first it may seem as if the two can never coexist, but eventually working out becomes part of an exciting, new healthy-way-of-life routine, and the effort to do it all becomes less daunting. Still, finding fitness in the chaos of motherhood has its challenges. Sometimes those challenges are only excuses. And, as you'll discover in the next secret, *there are no good excuses.*

MOM 2 MOM

I work part-time so I can be with my kids more, but when I need some solo miles I have no problem taking my youngest into day care. He loves it there so it's a win-win.

—Cindy, mom of three
Minneapolis, Minnesota

Secret Number Two

THERE ARE
NO GOOD EXCUSES

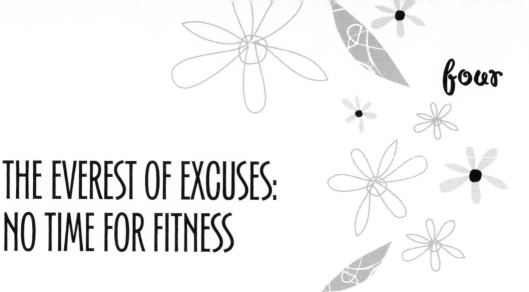

four

THE EVEREST OF EXCUSES: NO TIME FOR FITNESS

Ever feel like you're having a naughty, twisted love affair with Father Time? You love him, you hate him, you want him around, you wish he would leave you forever? With kids who amaze us in every way possible, it's hard not to look ahead to the future, to look back to the past. We can't wait to see our children mature, but we're sad to see them outgrow their first pair of toddler shoes.

With so much concern about the past and future, it's easy to forget about living in the present moment. It's the most difficult no-brainer in the world: All we have is *this* moment, the present. And it's that art of mindfulness that teaches you to turn your attention to the present moment, whether it's to gaze lovingly into your child's eyes or to work up a sweat. Learning how to make the most of each moment, being a mindful mama, is one of the basic skills of all fit moms.

But it's hard to live mindfully with time slipping through your hands. With twenty-four hours in a day, you'd think devoting just one hour to fitness would be a cinch. And yet time, or the lack thereof, is an uphill battle for all of us. But the struggle isn't insurmountable. Living in the moment isn't obsessing over a ticking clock. Don't let Father Time control you or give you an excuse to skip your workout, because, come on, will you ever have enough time?

Fit moms committed to getting their exercise work a little magic to factor it into their day. Along with a few tricks (we'll share those with you later), they make time, take time, share time, or snare time. And you can, too.

Make Time

We make time when we exercise while nothing else is vying for our attention. For many of us that means while we could be sleeping (or should be sleeping, ladies). Or, if you work in an office, you might skip your lunch hour (if you even take one). Up early, to bed late, go hungry. Your choice. You *make* the time to work out.

For many successfully fit moms, making time is the only surefire way to make fitness happen. You don't have to scrimp on sleep every night, but a few early morning workouts can ground a weekly fitness regimen. Whatever you set for your minimum requirements for exercise, consider making the time, because then nothing but you can keep you from your workout.

It sounds logical: Set the alarm two hours earlier and you're not taking time away from raising, nurturing, and protecting your family. You make it to work on time (even if your desk happens to be the kitchen table) and you don't sacrifice time with your partner, either.

But wait, it's not that simple. Let's factor in the rest of the story: You were up in the middle of the night to comfort your two-year-old and then let the dog outside for a quick pee; when you made it back to bed, you lay awake until 4 a.m., until your alarm rang at 5:30.

This is a true test of your determination. Do you roll out of bed before the sun rises to get in your workout? What will it be? A little more sleep or the triumph of a workout, cup of coffee, and shower before anyone else wakes up?

Take heed of sleep deprivation, though. Anecdotal evidence suggests a direct relationship between sleep and patience. Lack of sleep manifests itself as crabbiness, especially later in the day. However, if you want to see crabby, look for a fit mama who hasn't exercised for a week. Now that's crabby.

When you make time for a workout, measure the cost-benefit of lost sleep (or your lunch hour, if that's what you're losing). If you know the workout gained is more beneficial than whatever else you intended for your time, then go for it.

- When I first started running I could only get out after 10 p.m. There is only one streetlight near the house, so I mapped out 250 meters and ran back and forth under that light for thirty minutes.
- I've had to sleep in my running clothes so that I could get up at the crack of dawn to run before the kids woke up.
- I skip happy hour with my girlfriends.
- I work out over my lunch hour at work.
- When my youngest was born, I would nurse her at 3 a.m. and start my run at 4 a.m.
- I have canceled a meeting at work to get my workout in.

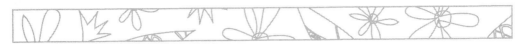

Take Time

Taking time requires that something gives, and usually requires the employ of child care: for example, hiring someone to watch the kids at home, keeping the kids at day care for an extra hour, or using the child care center at the gym. This might also include negotiating time with your partner. You *take* the time away from mothering to work out.

Taking time to work out can be the most personally satisfying (selfish?) option. Although this can be more costly (irresponsible?) due to the need to pay for child care, this becomes "free" (guilty?) time without children.

A mother should no more feel selfish, irresponsible, or guilty about her fitness goals than she should about good oral hygiene or preparing healthy meals. Exercising for our health reduces a host of chronic diseases, including heart disease, the number one killer of women. So is a woman who exercises selfish? Irresponsible? Guilty? How about *smart*?

Be sure you have enough sitters "on call" to make this a viable option. Having one good babysitter is important, but your fitness can't possibly rely on the availability of a single sitter. Build up your list when you don't need it so you're not in a panic when you do. (This method works well for date night and girls' night out, too.) Sharing a sitter among workout pals is a great way to share costs and get your kids excited about your workouts. Having friends to play with is a bonus for almost every kid—the kids probably won't even notice you've gone. Fellow Hot (Sweaty) Mamas also make good sitters. Take turns working out while you swap taking care of the kids.

Sure, there could be a few tangible downsides to deal with aside from the cash you part with if you pay for a sitter. These might include enduring the tantrum from a toddler in the midst of separation anxiety or the virus your child picked up at the gym's on-site child care center (which may prevent you from going back to the gym for a week or more). Again, measure the risks and benefits when deciding if you should take time for fitness. Sometimes it's the stolen moments that are the most energizing; this time feels closest to the "me time" you used to enjoy before children.

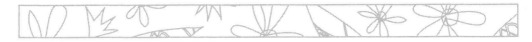

How Moms Take Time

- My husband takes the kids on an adventure every Saturday morning while I ride my bike.
- I paid my nanny two hours of overtime on Thanksgiving so I could get in a run.
- My husband and I both enjoy working out, and our weekends are that much better when we have a regular sitter. Babysitters who will work on Saturday or Sunday mornings are a must.
- My neighbor and I sometimes have "playdates" and take turns working out.
- I have begged/humiliated myself for child care.
- I've allowed my kids more video time so I can get in a treadmill workout.

Share Time

Mothers on a mission often find creative solutions that allow them to work out *with* their children. They *share* this time, together. We can only hope this is mutually satisfying. Jogging strollers, bike trailers, baby carriers that allow moms to "wear" their babies during workouts—this smells like quality time for fitness enthusiasts.

Make sure exercising with children is an option for you. That means acquiring whatever paraphernalia suits your exercise regimen. If you like to run, consider a treadmill for home use and/or a jogging stroller; cyclists may need a stationary trainer and/or a bike trailer; strength training might require some dumbbells and other props such as bands, balls, and kettlebells; for mind-body workouts, a good DVD player and a collection of yoga and Pilates videos will help. Do your homework first so you make a smart purchase. Give your friends' equipment a test drive and ask the store where you are shopping to let you give it a try before making the final selection. Such purchases can have a substantial price tag, but if you spend lots of quality time using the equipment, the investment is quickly amortized.

Sometimes sharing a workout with children isn't exactly the plan, it's more like Plan B— like when you sleep through your alarm or you can't find a sitter. Be proactive, not reactive when it comes to these detours in your day. If you haven't already, figure out how to include your children in your fitness routine. Consider pushing, pulling, or wearing the little ones and having older kids tag along however they are capable (think bike, scooter, roller skates).

This is easy, if they love it. If not, consider how you feel about exercising when you'd rather be on the couch reading a novel. You might start out sluggish, but once you get going you're glad you made the effort. Same mentality applies. Just get 'em going.

To prevent a mutiny, get creative and take your imagination on the move. This may or may not be what child psychologists had in mind for creative play, but turning your walk or run into a scavenger hunt or an hour-long game of "I Spy" just might put everyone in the mood for a workout. Always try to reward your kids for their good behavior during or after your workout. Finish at a local park or let them join you for the final stretch home.

Try as you might, your children may not be convinced that Mom's workouts are a good use of *their* time. Be prepared to bribe (candy, ice cream, video games, pretty much anything on the American Academy of Pediatrics' list of no-nos); negotiate for five more minutes, ten more minutes, or whatever you think they can tolerate; and when all hope is lost, set your sights on another day. Hey, you tried.

On those days when everything clicks, however, this brand of family fitness is worth it. Running in circles around the track can be more fun when your favorite little people are playing in the field or attempting to run "just like Mommy." On the bike, a destination ride to the home of a playmate or a beloved relative brings on a double-whammy adrenaline high from the satisfaction of a good multitasking sweat. A trip to the park can be as much of a workout for you as it is for your children, or you can conduct your own boot camp while kids play in the backyard. Pull out a jump rope and exercise band and put them to good use. Who says you can't pump iron while watching a Thomas the Train video? Secret Number Five has more strategies to include kids in your fitness routine.

How Moms Share Time

- When my son was a newborn, I'd hold him in my arms and do my salsa dance workout video. I did it almost daily when I was pregnant, and he seemed to instantly recognize the familiar movement and was soothed by it.
- I once did the elliptical for forty-five minutes while my youngest was in a Baby Björn. He was about eighteen pounds at the time—it was quite a workout!
- I've taken my kids with me and had them sit at the edge of the room while I worked out. It didn't go so well!
- I run my kids in the stroller, with the promise of park play at the end. Then at the park I push them on the swing while I do lunges and squats, then arm work on the monkey bars while they boot around.
- Yoga with my (naked) two-year-old jumping all over me. It was very relaxing (not).
- Baby tosses are always good—you know, squat with the baby and then toss him up into the air, catch him, and go back into a squat.

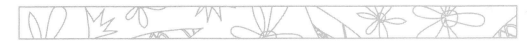

Snare Time

Our kids are masters of make-believe. You think they're sitting solemnly in church, only to find out they're pretending to be held prisoner in a castle full of evildoers. Maybe they just shared the wonderful realization that they can look at you, pretending to listen, while imagining you're a *Tyrannosaurus rex* that's grown a human head. Yep, kids turn the mundane into something fantastic. We should learn from them.

Sometimes, no matter how hard we try, there is simply no way to take, make, or share time. That's when we mamas have to be crafty, too. Figure out ways to turn those everyday activities into mini workouts. Get sneaky with your time and trap a workout.

Look for every opportunity to sneak in a mini workout. Sure, park your car at the far end of the lot, but pick it up a notch and walk briskly into work, the grocery store, or the doctor's office. Ask your coworkers to take meetings outside and discuss the agenda on a walk. The fresh air will spark creativity and add energy to the rest of your day. Are you meeting that friend you haven't seen in months? Instead of catching up over coffee, walk and talk on a trail or on side-by-side treadmills at a gym.

Anytime you're otherwise standing still is an opportunity to snare some fitness into your day. Waiting at the bus stop? Try some calf raises on the curb. Standing in line at the motor vehicles department? Take a number and do leg lifts until it's your turn to face the cranky lady behind the counter. Kids having fun playing in the bath? Keep an eye on them while you do tricep dips on the side of the tub.

You can also snare time for a workout while literally running errands in everyday life. Use that jogger or bike trailer to get to the dry cleaner, drugstore, or post office. Forget the courtesy shuttle—drop your car off for service and walk home. Sometimes it's possible to be double-booked. Run around the baseball field during your son's practice, or swim while your older kids hang out at the beach. While this may sound crazy, sometimes you have to be unorthodox to meet your goals.

Attack housework like a workout, too. Try moving from one activity to the next without taking breaks to make phone calls or grab a snack. In fact, set an alarm and aim to get certain tasks done before the bell rings. Clean with fervor. You'll get more done and get your heart rate up in the process. Consider buying a pair of those ankle weights your mom used to wear; they might look a little funny, but they'll take vacuuming to a whole new level. If you typically leave manual labor to the man in the house, talk to him about swapping weekend duties. Mowing the lawn, shoveling snow, and hauling garbage will do more for your fitness than sitting on the couch folding laundry (unless you're lunging and squatting as you fold, which we also recommend).

Look to your inner child for ideas on how you can take charge of your life and make a workout appear where it didn't exist before.

How Moms Snare Time

- Sit-ups while reading a story to my baby sitting on my stomach.
- I let my three-year-old lay draped across my back as I pulled weeds so I could further engage my core muscles and work my legs.
- I've done squats with baby in the Baby Björn carrier while cooking dinner.
- Sometimes my son has dinner in the stroller while I get a quick three miles in.
- Choosing between working out and grocery shopping for a last-minute dinner party, I decided to do both: I loaded my daughter in the bike trailer and rode to the grocery store.
- Squats in the shower while shampooing and conditioning!
- Walking on the treadmill during conference calls.

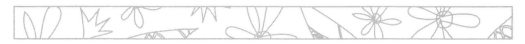

Most of us use a combination of make-time, take-time, share-time, and snare-time strategies to fold fitness into our day and avoid taxing any one area of life for the sake of a workout. If you're doing some of this already, you might not consciously think about acquiring your time for fitness in these ways. Labeling these tactics, though, makes your planning more deliberate and might help you find hidden opportunities to break a sweat.

In a perfect world, you get up early and nobody even knows you've been gone; stroller rides coincide with naptime; the sitter is their favorite person on the planet. No one cries. Everyone is happy. But sometimes (dare we say usually?) it isn't so perfect. Sometimes the kids wake up just as you're leaving; sometimes you're pushing a rolling temper tantrum; sometimes they just want you to stay with them. Do you? No. Let them cry and consider it "Ferberizing" for fit moms. Kids need to learn early on (or eventually) that, just as there are certain times in the day for sleep, there are also times in the day for exercise. They may not always like it, but you are taking steps to establish fitness as a family value.

Four Time Tricks for Fit Moms

Looking for that twenty-fifth hour? You can't create any extra time in your day, but you can become more efficient with those precious moments you do have. Give the following time-saving tactics a try—they just might give birth to that hour you need for fitness.

Time Trick Number One: Give a Little to Get a Little

We're talking about time here. As a mom, you're on call 24/7, so it might be hard to imagine giving more time to your kids. If you're a stay-at-home mom, you definitely think we're crazy. But we're not talking about the half-assed attempts of playing "Go Fish" while preparing dinner or reading Dr. Seuss while checking e-mail. Sometimes you need to stop multitasking. Try committing spans of at least twenty minutes to play. Saturating your kids with "mom time" will give them their fill so you can have an hour without hearing "Mommy!" After a mutually satisfying play session you will spend less time running back and forth, say from your exercise video to the playroom, and less mental energy fearing you're not being the best mom you can be.

Time Trick Number Two: Become a Pack Rat

Despite the alarming reproductive cycle of kid clutter, resist the urge to get rid of all those excess toys. Instead, place a small arsenal in strategic locations. An old laundry basket that contains a big beach towel or blanket, sand toys, and sports balls works well in the back of the car for a stop at the track or outdoor tennis court. A small child's backpack with books sits easily in the bottom of the jogger. While you're packing up, keep an inventory of suckers, snacks, and juice boxes for emergency consumption. If you have a kid who is still in diapers, keep changing essentials in these places, too (and stashed in your car).

MOM 2 MOM

I keep a "just in case" bag packed with sneakers, running gear, and swimming gear—just in case I have an hour that I hadn't counted on to get an extra workout in. It makes life easier to adjust plans, and it decreases excuses!

—Gretchen, mom of two
Guilderland, New York

Time Trick Number Three: Be Overprepared

Remember to keep yourself ready, too. Find an old gym bag (or two) and keep them stocked with workout essentials and toiletries. Anything you would use to get ready at home, clone for your gym bag. Hoarding a bra in there (or any item you would not want to be without) will come in handy. Old sneakers do have a life in your trunk for those days when—whoops!—you forgot to pack them in your bag. All this packing might seem overzealous, but it can translate into an extra fifteen minutes for a snared workout.

Time Trick Number Four: Location, Location, Location

Drive time eats away at your workout, or cuts into some other part of your life. If you have to drive twenty minutes before you even start your workout, then you're burning precious time. Working out at home is ideal when it comes to cutting travel time, but if you belong to a gym, make sure it's close by. Chart routes for exercising from home that don't require you to drive to a workout destination.

Now it's time for you to work some magic and apply these time tricks to your own life. We know, it sounds easy on paper—where everything is black and white. Real life is shades of gray, and excuses lurk in the shadows. In the next chapter we'll shed some light on distinguishing between excuses and reasons.

MOM 2 MOM

I hate to take—and often don't have—the time it takes to drive to the gym. But I can use the fifty "me" minutes before my daughter gets off the bus to run four miles and stretch before meeting her on the corner. It's a perfect fit and removes any burden to exercise.

—Kate, mom of two
Minneapolis, Minnesota

five

ERADICATE EXCUSES

MOM 2 MOM

Excuses, excuses, excuses. As a parent you've likely heard some doozies from your kids—why they don't want to take a bath or why they can't possibly go to bed. The older ones craft excuses to justify being out past curfew or why their bedrooms resemble toxic waste sites. Making excuses is, simply put, a defense mechanism we learn at a very early age and an art we perfect as we get older.

With years of excuse-making experience behind us, justifying even the most unhealthy and illogical choices is easy. On the surface, excuses seem harmless. Like a well-placed throw rug, they prevent us from seeing the dirt that's underneath. Excuses make us appear more whole and well-adjusted than we really are. Excuses are nothing more than little tiny lies we tell ourselves. Sometimes they are so good even *we* believe them.

Excuses build up in our system like a silent poison. They sully our attitude and outlook on life. Eventually our minds become as toxic as that teenager's bedroom. It's time to clean up your mindset, because all of those excuses are keeping you from doing what's truly important.

There are things you start believing when you have a child with a disability. You start making up things you'll never do and your kids will never do. And you *are* making it up. Most of these excuses cut off the abilities in their lives and your own. Before having kids we loved to hike, bike, and camp. But after having a child with cerebral palsy and spina bifida, we told ourselves we couldn't do those things anymore. Then we were left sitting at home watching television. We decided it's only true if we let it be true. We started asking ourselves: What if we hike with her on our back? What if we get a jogging stroller? Now my husband and I fight to carry Lucy. Now we ask ourselves: What can we do next?

—Rachel, mom of two
Salt Lake City, Utah

Start by making your mind a Superfund site; spend a little mental currency and decontaminate.

Learn how to differentiate reasons from excuses. Reasons exist in reality. In the realm of not exercising, reasons are plentiful. Sometimes, truly, you are better served forgoing that workout. You know you have a good reason to skip the workout when you feel relief after making the decision. That's because reasons hold weight, substance. Reasons are a positive force in decision making.

Excuses, by contrast, are negative and, if applied, leave you with negative afterthoughts (typically manifesting as guilt). When you make an excuse, there's a nagging voice that leaves you unsatisfied with your decision.

The last time you skipped a workout, was it a reason or an excuse?

Reasons are succinct; excuses take explaining.
Reasons don't leave room for second-guessing; excuses do.
Reasons are truth; excuses are half-truths at best.
Reasons don't crumble on examination; excuses do.
Reasons are not driven by fear; excuses are.
Reasons allow us to reach our potential; excuses help us cheat.

The next time you consider opting out of exercise, stop yourself before you make an excuse. ACT on it:

Analyze your attitude. What are you thinking or feeling that's keeping you from forging full steam ahead?

Consider the circumstances. Now deal with the facts: What is really impinging on your workout?

Think it through. Are you reacting to a reason or an excuse? Are you left with relief or guilt?

Here are five case studies demonstrating ways to ACT on fitness and excuse-proof your workouts.

1. I'm too tired to exercise.

Analyze your attitude: Being a mom is a tiring endeavor that can make you more inclined to hit the hay than hit the gym.

Consider the circumstances: If you're a new mom waking every few hours with the baby, or if you have pushed your body to the limit with sleep deprivation for another reason, you may have crossed the line from tired to fatigued. Fatigue can definitely have harmful effects on our health. But more often than not it is our brain wanting us to conserve energy; our brain is like our grandma who wants us to eat a little bit more and sit and rest a spell on her comfortable couch. "*Don't overdo it!*" our brain says, in well-meaning protection.

Think it through: Indeed, sleep is important, particularly while caring for a newborn. Erring on the side of sleep while your body heals and you adjust to new motherhood is valid. And more rest is justified if you are so sleep deprived you can't function at work or home. But not wanting to roll out of bed when your alarm rings? Feeling that afternoon slump? Sorry. Deal with it. Our need for sleep doesn't end when our kids grow out of that newborn stage. In fact, the need for more sleep seems to grow right along with our children. Often the best way to combat fatigue involves lacing up your gym shoes. A little exercise will not contribute to the energy drain you feel. On the contrary, exercise plugs up that drain. If you're feeling pooped (and that's different from exhausted), moving will stimulate both mind and body, helping you feel more alert and, dare we say, spunky.

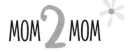

Excuse-proof your workout: If you feel the excuse "I'm too tired to exercise" coming on, defend your workout in stages. Stage one: Tell yourself you're only going to put on your exercise clothes. You'll make the decision to work out after you're dressed. Stage two: You're dressed; you might as well do something. You don't have to do much; even ten minutes will rev up your energy level. Stage three: With ten minutes under your belt you can decide whether or not to continue. Sometimes fatigue will win out here, but that's fine; you still exercised. Sometimes ten minutes

> After my triplets were born I hired a nanny to come to the house to help me during the day. I know I should have been napping during that time to store up the energy to get me through the long nights, but nope—I found energy to work out for an hour and I'm sure glad I did!
>
> —Linda, mom of three
> Falmouth, Maine

is enough to make you realize you wanted that workout more than you wanted to create an indentation on the couch.

2. Working out is for Super Mom down the street.

Analyze your attitude: Would you just look at her? She does it all, including regular exercise, with such ease and grace. She doesn't dress like a slob and even on her worst hair day she looks cute. To make matters worse, she's nice, so you can't even hate her. How could you live with the stress of pursuing that ideal?

Consider the circumstances: The truth of the matter is you can never know what it takes for another woman to do anything she does. And we're betting whatever Super Mom is achieving, it's hardly with ease and grace. Besides, there is no point in comparing yourself to others; that's a distraction from focusing on you and what you can accomplish with your life.

Think it through: Don't underestimate yourself. You are just as equipped to achieve your goals as anyone else. Focus on what you are doing, what you can do, and what you want to do. In this case, feeling inadequate is *never* a reason to skip a workout.

Excuse-proof your workout: If you really think Super Mom's got something you don't, ask her how she does it. Odds are she'll tell you it takes some serious juggling and coordinating for her to stay fit, too, but maybe you'll glean a new tip or two. Better yet, ask her if you can join her in a workout.

MOM 2 MOM

I know a younger friend and newer mom who is able to work a full-time job on night shifts, be in the navy reserves, teach fitness classes at the gym, and still run half marathons. It makes my whines about being too tired to run seem ridiculous.

—Rachel, mom of two
Frederick, Maryland

3. Personal trainers are for people in Hollywood.

Analyze your attitude: Look at the way tabloids flaunt the taut tummies of movie-star moms; hoisting their baby on one skinny hip, their biceps rippling just enough to produce envy. You already know better not to compare yourself with these moms. Still, this brand of fitness is easy to dismiss; they have hired help, after all.

Consider the circumstances: Anyone who spends time in a gym will tell you that personal trainers are becoming more and more commonplace. And it's not just for Hollywood stars. Everyday people of all abilities are seeking out qualified professionals to help educate and motivate them to achieve their personal best. Trainers meet with clients on a regular basis to discuss their fitness goals and develop a realistic plan to achieve them. But perhaps the most important thing a trainer does is provide the push to get you moving for the right reasons. Likewise, they can help you eradicate excuses.

Think it through: No matter how much you pay a personal trainer, she can't do the work for you. Sure, those movie-star moms pay a significant sum for someone to tell them how to work out, but they still have to sweat. There are too many low-cost or no-cost fitness options out there to make affordability an excuse to forgo fitness. In order to keep cost from being a reason to avoid workouts, you have to make fitness affordable (or free).

Excuse-proof your workout: You need to sweat, but not necessarily over the cost of a personal trainer. Consider splitting a training session with a friend or two. But you don't even have to step foot inside a gym. All you need is a good fitness mentor, someone who is doing what you'd like to do. Turn to a sports league or club. Find a friend who can share his/her knowledge and help you devise a motivating plan that works for you. Look to the Internet for training blogs and Web sites (check out the appendix for a list of resources), download workouts to your iPod, track progress on your smart phone. Yes, there's an app for that.

MOM **2** MOM

My friend Shannon is extremely dedicated and consistently exercises. We trained for a half marathon together even though we live six hours apart. She would send me fitness gear and music from her iTunes library. She keeps me motivated.

—Heather, mom of two
Evansville, Indiana

4. I don't like to work out.

Analyze your attitude: For starters, it makes you breathe hard. It can be uncomfortable. It causes perspiration, smears makeup, wilts hair, and produces residual soreness.

Consider the circumstances: Perhaps you were scarred for life after a terrifying incident on the playground. Maybe going to phys-ed class made you break out in hives. If you were the last kid standing while picking teams or you felt like you were a gangly adolescent that looked as awkward as you felt playing sports, then you might still be hanging on to angst of yesteryear. If someone even so much as suggested you weren't a natural athlete or good at a certain sport, you might have falsely accepted that and made it part of "who you are" and so you no longer associate anything that makes you sweat with something that is fun or empowering.

Think it through: We bet you're not a big fan of gynecologist appointments and pap smears, either. You probably wouldn't skip your yearly checkup—it's too risky to neglect your health, right? Consider fitness another regular appointment for your health. Can you put the past behind you? Is it possible to find an activity you like to do—at least a little? No one should be forced to do anything they don't like, but there are too many ways to exercise to use this as an excuse.

Excuse-proof your workout: If you really disdain exercise, consider a team activity or join a group that keeps exercise social. You may not ever love to exercise, but you'll have another good reason to do it. Picking teams, as adults, isn't nearly as stressful.

5. Family always comes first.

Analyze your attitude: Someone always needs you, right? You're too important to steal away time for something as self-indulgent as exercise.

Consider the circumstances: Last we checked you're a member of the family, too. If you're a member of the family, and family comes first, then you deserve a little time on the top of the podium. Likewise, if it's important to "be there"

MOM 2 MOM

When I finally found a doctor that was able to diagnose my chronic disease and help me manage it, I knew it was time to make drastic changes to support my treatment. A quote jumped out at me from *You: Staying Young* by Michael F. Roizen, MD, and Mehmet C. Oz, MD, that says: "Human cells have a fitness memory of about three years. So, amazingly, if you adopt a fit lifestyle now, within three years, your body will behave as if you've been fit your entire life." I made the change two years ago. I have done several 5Ks and 10Ks and a half marathon, and I am going through the certification process to become a Pilates instructor. My current Pilates instructor has referred to me as an athlete. *An athlete!* I can hardly wait to see what that third year brings and to know that soon, my cells won't know anything other than their "owner" as an athlete!

—Amy, mom of two
Burnsville, Minnesota

for your family, then it's all the more important that you find the time to exercise. You'll live and "be there" a lot longer for your loved ones.

Think it through: Unless you're going way overboard, neglecting your duties as a mother and spouse to fit in excessive workouts, then "putting family first" is only an excuse to avoid exercise. Sure, there will come a time when you have a good reason to skip a workout so that you can tend to your family, but used excessively this excuse can be a familiar crutch.

Excuse-proof your workout: Just remember, you'll be a better mom if you take time for yourself. Also, every time you exercise you are setting a good example for your children, who are more likely to grow up fit if they have parents who exercise.

The way you feel after exercise far exceeds the relief you think you feel when you skip a workout. Work out and you get stronger. Overcome an excuse and you develop strength in other ways. You stand taller, breathe deeper, and develop more integrity as you make a conscious effort to be true to yourself. Overcome an excuse just once and you take away its power; the excuse becomes easier to dismiss the next time.

We could fill this book with all the lame excuses we use to avoid exercise. We don't want to write that book and you certainly don't want to read it. Using the excuse-busting examples above, you should now be equipped to eradicate any excuses that come your way. The next chapter will help you sharpen the personal qualities that will carry you through the tough times—attributes that will help you rise above those excuses and conquer your workouts.

MOM 2 MOM

After my husband sustained a back injury the physical therapist prescribed weights and cardio exercise three times a week. We made sure he got that exercise for about three years. After a while it dawned on me that if we could make room for him to exercise because of his health, then we could make room for me to exercise for my health. That's what it took. I started at just twice a week and never did less than that ever again.

—Erin, mom of four
Minneapolis, Minnesota

Don't let the perfect be the enemy of the good. I always tell myself if I didn't get one thing done, I can always do something else. If I didn't make it to my spinning class, I can take a walk. If I didn't make it to my strength class, I can lift dumbbells at home.

—Carrie, mom of one
Hurst, Texas

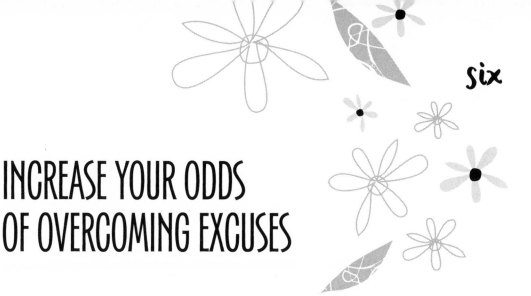

six

INCREASE YOUR ODDS OF OVERCOMING EXCUSES

By now you have what it takes to be *that* woman. *That* woman who appears (at least on the outside) to manage it all and fit in her workouts. Super Mom doesn't have anything over you. Your power is in your character. Leap tall buildings in a single bound? No. But honing certain attributes will give you more power over your time and those villainous excuses.

Cultivating Your Character

Life certainly gets more interesting with age. We spend more time thinking about the person we are and the person we want to become. As you do, think about the following personality traits. These characteristics exist within you (some more than others) and can give you the edge you need to fit fitness into your day. Odds are, developing these characteristics will positively impact all aspects of your life—in and out of your gym clothes.

Adaptability allows you to adjust to changing circumstances. It involves making changes to your schedule as well as to your attitude about what's going on around you. It's crucial to finding time and using it

MOM 2 MOM

I find that I have to operate with a Plan B ready for those days that the kids wake up with a fever, or have to stay home from school, or just need me. I keep a huge folder of workouts and if I can't get to the gym during the day, I'll either pull something out and do it at home, or wait until after "Tuck-in Time" to get my workout in.

—Whitney, mom of three
Winter Springs, Florida

efficiently. Sure, it's nice to have a routine, but don't become a slave to it. When opportunities present themselves . . . *pounce*! For instance, keep your gym bag packed in your car, even on days you don't plan to work out. When your meeting gets canceled or Dad wants to pick up the kids from school, that's your opportunity to head to the gym. Be prepared both physically and mentally to embrace the situation. It's time to become spontaneous again.

Initiative is taking that first step toward whatever goal you are pursuing. It's vital to making the most of your time. Having the gym bag packed in the car is one thing. Working out rather than hitting happy hour is another. What you want to accomplish doesn't happen on its own. As you already know, time is precious. How do you want to spend your time? (Remember, no one else is going to get fit for you.)

Confidence is a belief in yourself and your actions. Being confident in your choices will help you protect your interests. Sure, if you bail on happy hour you will miss out on a few good laughs. But remember you're doing what is important to you. What is *really* going to give you a "happy hour"? Make that choice and don't look back.

Persistence keeps you going. Actually, it's just the proper way of being pigheaded. Just because you missed your 6 a.m. workout doesn't mean all is lost. Do not take a shower. Do not coif your hair. Keep those gym shorts on, girlfriend. At the very least, at the end of the day you'll look like you worked out. If you're heading to an office or other obligation that requires you shower, be stubborn,

MOM 2 MOM

I think it's important to have workout clothes that are cute enough that you don't mind wearing them 24/7. If my morning run gets delayed, I can be ready to run any time throughout the day at a moment's notice. I keep running shoes in my car so I can wear a pair of sandals or casual shoes the rest of the time. I also use a little bit of tinted moisturizer and brown mascara. I put it on every time I get out of the shower so I always have a little bit of makeup on. I think of this as my uniform. But I always feel cute and I am always ready to run. Like having a superpower.

—Stephanie, mom of two
Pleasant View, Tennessee

I love the relaxing hours of early evening when everything is winding down. Short term, that surrender would feel good; but in the big picture I know I'm happiest after I've "taken care of business," and taken care of me.

—Laurie

nonetheless. Chances are, if you remain at the ready—if only mentally—you'll find an opportunity to squeeze in that workout. (See Adaptability, Initiative and Confidence, above.)

Creativity is the ability to transcend rules and the status quo in order to find a new path of your own. Creativity allows persistence to pay off. When you miss your morning workout—perhaps the only planned time you have for fitness—use your creative talents to reorganize or reengineer your day. Sometimes it takes a little ingenuity to take time, make time, share time, or snare time. Your options are not always obvious.

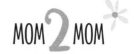

Last Resort

As crafty as we may become at eradicating excuses, it can boil down to a few mind games to get you out the door. Consider those cute new yoga pants you bought last week. You might miraculously find time to work out so that you have a good reason to wear them.

Yes, it sounds stupid and shallow. Yet, it *is* worth mentioning. If you look good, you feel good. You may not always need this superficial boost. Sometimes though, a brand-new performance tee or athletic skirt can, in fact, motivate you to drop whatever it is you're doing or plan to do and work up a sweat.

Perhaps you think your money—and motivation—is better spent on a race entry fee. Committing to a race holds you responsible to a certain amount of training. Suddenly, you are accountable for getting to the finish. Heck, now you're accountable for getting to the start.

Whatever it takes. Maybe it's the lure of a postworkout pancake breakfast, the reward of a pedicure, or just knowing you

I have a long history of being motivated by "something new." I have always been more eager to work out because of some new piece of apparel or workout gadget, as far back as childhood when I was certain each brand-new pair of sneakers would make me run faster.

—Kara

get to gab with your favorite workout pal. Figure out how best to bribe yourself into a workout. Whatever that is, whatever in the end gets you out the door, *that's* your secret weapon.

Above all, remember this: Bodies in motion stay in motion. Just turn on your autopilot and get through the business of being fit. Sure, you'll still face bumps in the road now and then but, as you know by now, there is usually a way around them. (Be sure to check the appendix for the "Sweaty Decision Tree" for when you're flummoxed about whether or not to workout.)

Next up: Common questions about living a fit life that, if left unaddressed, can send us on a detour away from the road to fitness.

The Excuse Buster Training Plan

Exercises in Adaptability

Lose your schedule for a day. Forget your routine and play things by ear. Maybe even let the kids help you decide what your plans are. Who knows, you may discover better solutions to managing your time.

Before you say "no," consider "yes." Saying no can protect your priorities, but sometimes saying yes in the right circumstances can take care of the time crunch by exposing you to a new, more efficient solution.

Exercises in Initiative

Make the first move. Some of us would never get out the door if our exercise partners didn't coordinate workouts. Next time, don't wait for an invitation; pick up the phone.

Plan ahead. Knowing what you physically want to do for a workout isn't enough. The logistics of staying fit are part of the workout. If you'll need child care, arrange it in advance. Make sure your partner knows your intentions so there are no questions or conflicts.

Exercises in Confidence

Educate. If your mother suggests you forgo your workout, don't crumble. Now is the perfect opportunity to explain just why it is you do what you do. We all have our own reasons for staying fit, but we share at least one: It makes us happy. Make sure the people who care about you know.

Walk away. There are some people who will never understand your devotion to fitness. Identify who those people are and know when it's not worth your effort to "show them the light."

Exercises in Persistence

Forget "forget it." Sure, sometimes your body needs a day to recover, but unless you've planned a day of rest don't let yourself off the hook so easily.

Make a list. Every time you skip a workout, write down what is keeping you from exercise. Then, take a look at your list and determine if you have a lame excuse or a legitimate reason.

Exercises in Creativity

Act like a kid. What are your children playing right now? Chances are you can turn their child's play into your workout. Hit the monkey bars, play tag, go skating.

Think like a kid. Imagine life with no limits. No rules, no time constraint, and money is no object. What do you want to do? Decide what it is before getting mired down on how to make it happen.

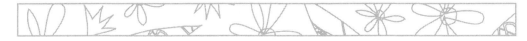

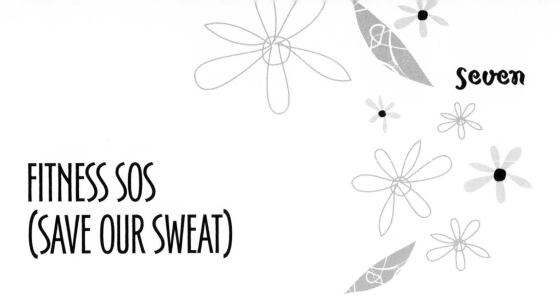

Seven

FITNESS SOS (SAVE OUR SWEAT)

Getting and keeping the momentum to stay fit takes work. As we discussed in the previous chapters, it can be hard to overcome the temptation to make an excuse whenever you just don't *feel* like exercising. This is especially true when you're stressed out, tired, or feeling a little lazy. The temptation is compounded when you're vexed with fitness conundrums. Even when your motivation is in the right place and obstacles appear, it's hard to know whether to go over them, under them, or around them. What to do? How to keep going? Should you even try?

Ignorance is not bliss, nor is it an excuse to skip a workout. In this Q&A chapter, we'll provide answers to common fitness questions that can stump even the most motivated moms. When questions like these are left unanswered, you might feel inclined to wave a white flag. Don't surrender your fitness goals. This chapter may be the flotation device that keeps your goals from sinking.

I'm Working Out; Why Can't I Lose Weight?

First, remember: Being a fit mom isn't the same as being a skinny mom. We all come in different shapes and sizes. While some of us will never be skinny, every one of us can be fit.

Sometimes those pounds aren't all bad. Because muscle weighs more than fat, the scale can fib a little. Instead of looking at the scale, take note of how your clothes fit. Tightening that belt a bit more? Odds are you're on the right track.

If you need to jump off the bed in order to get into your jeans, you might want to analyze the eating and exercise equation. This is especially so if you tend to "reward yourself" after a day of exercise. You might burn up to a thousand calories in a given workout—the equivalent of a Burger King Whopper and a small order of French fries. An hour of hard work destroyed in one greasy sitting. If fast food is not on your list of quick stops, don't assume you're in the clear. Too much snacking on healthy foods can do it, too.

Another culprit could be that you're not eating enough. Too few calories—especially if you're exercising—could set your body into "starving" mode. Your body will not want to shed that weight if it isn't being properly nourished. To be sure you're not leaning too far one way or the other, track your food intake in a diary so you'll know if you're "breaking even" or being underserved. A good online tool for this is Livestrong's MyPlate (http://www.livestrong.com/myplate).

It's possible you're doing everything right nutritionally; it's your workouts that need to be tweaked. If you exercise at one speed and one speed only, your body may need you to rev the gas up a bit, get your motor running. Work out a little harder on some days—increase your pace or decrease your rest time—or sprinkle your workout with some intervals to challenge your body to burn up more calories in short bursts. If you work out with a heart-rate monitor, know what your various training zones are, so you can alternate between fat-burning workouts and workouts that increase your level of fitness. (Learn more about heart-rate training online or check out *The Heart Rate Monitor Guidebook to Heart Zone Training* by Sally Edwards, Heart Zones Publishing, 2010.)

Also, every woman over twenty should be engaged in strength training to offset the inevitable bone loss that occurs with age. Another added benefit of muscle mass is that it increases metabolism; muscles are a more efficient calorie burner than fat.

I've Been at This Awhile; Why Am I Not Improving?

Logging tons of miles on the treadmill, but not getting any faster? Spending lots of time on your bike, but find your favorite route still takes the same amount of time? No doubt you've hit a plateau, but don't worry, there is a way off it.

If your workouts are on autopilot, it's time to take back the wheel. When your body becomes accustomed to doing the same workout, at the same intensity, for the same amount of time, it stops "reacting" to the exercise. Basically most exercise is designed to break down the body a little bit, so that during recovery your body knits itself together even stronger. If you don't push it, there's no breakdown, and then there are no gains in performance.

So mix up your workouts. You can still partake in your favorite flavor of exercise, just sample other types and intensities, too. Try a new cardiovascular or weight-lifting activity once a week. If you typically walk or run, get on a bike or try a cycling class. It's also important to vary the intensity of your workouts. You need to cross-train between forms of exercise as well as within them. If you're on that treadmill, try increasing the speed for two-minute intervals or increase the elevation. Mark certain days of the week as easy (recovery) days when your intensity level is lower. Then be sure to squeeze in some days of hard effort (push yourself close to breathlessness). And remember, too, to vary the duration of your workouts, so that you increase your endurance.

I'm Burned Out—How Can I Get Excited About My Workouts Again?

First, take a look at your routine. As in the example above, if you're doing the same workout day after day, burnout is inevitable. As we'll point out in the next secret, total fitness includes more than just cardiovascular work. The other four fit principles are flexibility, muscular endurance, muscular strength, and body composition. We also outline five additional fitness components that should be part of various workouts. If you're making an effort to address these, you'll find it difficult to be bored.

In addition to varying your workout, it's important to recover adequately from workouts by getting enough rest on a daily basis as well as in between workouts. While we're all for ingenious ways to schedule workouts, exercise doesn't have to happen every day. You should consider dedicating one day each week to resting your body and mind.

One good way to mix up your routine is to change your environment. If you typically work out indoors, get outside. Find a buddy to exercise with, too. Not only will the company fight boredom, but also you'll be privy to their workouts, which can expand your routine.

I'm Feeling a Little Sick—Should I Still Exercise?

When you're feeling under the weather, the best medicine is sometimes a little sweat. Studies out of the American College of Sports Medicine reveal that a little exercise can help lick a mild illness, such as a cold, faster. If you've got a case of the sniffles, a tickle in your throat, or a headache coming on—basically symptoms above the neck—go ahead and squeeze in that workout. The main tip here is to cut your intensity to half of what you would normally do. If after ten minutes you start to feel better (we're betting you do) then go on about your workout as you normally would. If not, keep your intensity and duration low.

Remember, too, that stress has an amazing way of manifesting itself physically. Sometimes, just getting out there to relieve the stress will melt away those sundry ailments.

Use common sense, though. If you're coming down with something and know your coworker was recently out sick with strep throat or your son was up vomiting last night, it's probably time to lay off and rest. If you've got a fever, consider that your pass to take a day off of exercise.

Will I Always Be This Sore?

There are two flavors of muscle soreness. The first is a kind of sore that reminds you that you are on a fitness mission. It does not leave you sidelined for days. Living a fit lifestyle does involve some level of discomfort. Whenever you make changes to your routine (which you should do if you want to continue to develop) you should notice a little discomfort. It means you're challenging yourself. Soon enough, your body will adapt. And that's when you know you need to make changes again. Yes, you must invite the soreness back. Our recommendation? A good soak in a bath of Epsom salt (sure, your kids may end up in the tub with you, but the soak will still do its job). Another fantastic remedy is regular massage. You don't have to see a masseuse for this. You'd be surprised at how adept little hands and feet are at kneading tight muscles.

The second kind of muscle soreness may more accurately be described as pain. Are you left unable to bend over and tie your own shoes? Perhaps you can't pick up your toddler without grimacing in pain. Whatever the problem, if you can't perform your daily tasks, you are likely overdoing it a bit. But don't let that little twinge in your foot, that tight hamstring, or the hot spot on your heel be a temptation for you *not* to work out.

However, it's important to address the twinges and tight spots before they become full-blown injuries. Make sure your fitness program balances your body and helps prevent injury.

My (Fill in the Blank) Hurts—Should I Back Off?

When soreness develops into inflammation it's important to enlist two important remedies: ice and the nonsteroidal anti-inflammatory of your choice. Keep gel packs in your freezer (we recommend the kind already inserted in an Ace-type bandage to wrap around the aching body part). Sometimes a few days of ice and anti-inflammatories can do the trick. Also, be sure footwear and equipment fit correctly.

Meanwhile, you may need to take a day or two off, or back off from the intensity or duration to allow your body to get back on track. When you're ready to resume your workouts, don't start where you left off; return to fitness gradually.

In some cases the remedy for the pain is more exercise. If a muscle imbalance is causing overuse or injury, it's important to strengthen the slacking muscles.

Sometimes it's a mobilizer muscle, such as the abductor muscle on the outside of the leg, that doesn't have enough support from its stabilizer muscle, in this case the adductors on the inside of the leg. This might cause pain in your hip or knee. Go ahead and stand on one foot to test the balance between your abductors and adductors. Still standing? If not, you likely need to strengthen the muscles in the inner thighs.

Other times the imbalance is in how we use our muscles. For example, if you spend six hours a day hunched over a keyboard and no time with your arms behind you, the muscles that pull your arms in front of you will become tighter. This may not be a huge problem while you're sitting at your desk, but once you take up your favorite sport and engage those underused and weaker muscles, your position and technique will suffer, and you risk injury. In this case, or if you participate in a sport that favors a certain set of muscles, spend time strengthening the underused muscles.

If discomfort or pain persists, call in the experts. We can't give you a deadline for this; you have to go with your gut when it comes to seeking medical attention. Depending on your ailment, you might benefit from the help of a physical therapist, chiropractor, or sports medicine doctor. Not sure where to start? Check with your family doc to get direction, or get recommendations from your workout partners.

Should I Work Out in This Weather?

When the weather doesn't cooperate with your exercise plans, you have two alternatives: head indoors or toughen up. If you're accustomed to enjoying nature's beauty while working out, you probably aren't excited about sweating indoors. Consider watching television, listening to music, or reading a magazine to entertain your mind while you work out on equipment. A group fitness class is another indoor option.

If you don't have any indoor exercise alternatives, prepare for the weather. In cold temps, dress in layers with water-wicking fabrics against your skin. Wear a hat to keep the heat in. Be assured, if the desire is there, you'll find gear to protect you from whatever temperature you're willing to face.

In warm weather, drink plenty of water and stay hydrated. Use sunscreen with an SPF of at least 15. Remember that dark colors attract the sun, so dress "whitely" and lightly. If you can, time your workout for the cooler part of the day—early in the morning or late at night—and look for sprinklers to hit along the way.

Should I Eat Now or Wait Until After My Workout?

When it comes to what and how much to eat before a workout, we have one suggestion: trial and error. This is one area where everyone is different. Depending on how long your workout is, and how long it's been since you last ate, you may want to eat something before you start. If you get up early to exercise it's especially important to replenish your energy stores after a good night's rest, otherwise you may literally be "running on empty."

Good choices for stomach-friendly foods include bananas, peanut butter and jelly toast, yogurt, or a small glass of juice. Again, try different food alternatives to see what works best for you.

I Know This Is Good for Me, But Do I Look as Silly as I Feel?

Don't think you fit the mold for the perfect fit mom? Does anyone? There really is no such thing. Nope, we come in all shapes, sizes, and abilities.

If you find it easy to feel inspired by others but uneasy about your own efforts, be patient; that confidence will come. The purpose of going to a gym isn't to compare yourself with others. Truly, people at the gym are more interested in getting in their own workouts than critiquing yours. Don't worry about how you look; celebrate the fact that you're doing it. Besides, this fitness journey of yours is about continually trying new things. You'll never be good at everything. You are better off looking silly (and laughing at yourself) while living life more fully than doing nothing at all.

I Lost My Training Partner; Now What Do I Do?

If you are accustomed to working out with someone else and that someone is no longer part of the training plan, you are left holding the torch on your own. Finding the motivation and will to work out without a faithful partner may not be easy at first, but once you dig around inside to figure out why it is you need to sweat, you'll realize all the good reasons are yours and yours alone.

No doubt, having friends to motivate you (especially for early morning workouts) is a boon to your fitness, but they can become crutches, too. Hold yourself to workouts, even when your pals can't be there. Test your fitness faith by scheduling some solo workouts so you know who's got your back. You might discover you enjoy the solitude. And, no one's stopping you from finding a new workout partner. They're out there—go get 'em!

We hope this chapter has been the fitness preserver you need to save your sweat and drown out excuses for good. With your fitness afloat it's time to move on. The focus of Secret Number Three is your body: how to honor it so you feel as fit as you look.

Secret Number Three

BE AS GOOD TO
YOUR BODY
AS YOU ARE TO
YOUR CHILDREN

eight

GET MOVING: THERE'S MORE THAN ONE WAY TO EXERCISE

This whole book is about fitness as a lifestyle, but in this chapter we'll help you see that there is more depth and breadth to exercise than you may have considered. If all you're after is a hardcore sweat, you're missing out on other opportunities that will help you achieve total fitness. Understanding that fitness is multidimensional is the first step toward integrating fitness into your life, not just your day.

Being a Hot (Sweaty) Mama doesn't mean that exercise *always* has to make you hot and sweaty. Hard work can legitimize the time we reserve for working out, but when we are short-changed on time and energy, what we want isn't always what we get.

When a workout doesn't go as planned or doesn't happen at all, half of our brain says, "Be realistic." The other half says, "Try harder." This banter affects women who are struggling to get to the gym three times a week as well as those training for a marathon. Sometimes we can be a

> Being more accepting of what I *can* do instead of beating myself up for what I *don't* do has been, as you might expect, a positive, life-changing shift in mindset. After my third daughter was born I remember feeling like a fraction of my old self. I wasn't training for triathlons, but I was out walking with a baby in a front carrier and pushing the twins in a double jogging stroller (while walking the dog). I kept reminding myself I was still doing more than the majority of sedentary America.
>
> —Kara

little too hard on ourselves, even when we make the best, most realistic choice based on the time and energy available. What's worse, listening to those conflicting voices in our heads can hack away at our self-esteem or leave us feeling exhausted. It's time to ease up and give credit for the things we can accomplish.

Along with a personal treaty to feel content with whatever workouts you can squeeze in (remember you learned the difference between reasons and excuses in chapter 5), it helps to expand your options for exercise to include more than just one type of workout. This way, you have a Plan B if one doesn't work out. And diversifying your workouts is good for you—our bodies crave diversity of movement and it's vital to achieving total health and fitness.

> I started practicing yoga to help slow my mind and relieve anxiety, but when touching my toes became a monumental achievement, I realized it wasn't just my psyche that was out of balance—it was my body, too.
>
> —Laurie

The Anatomy of Fitness

When planning your workouts, or perhaps feeling depressed about a lack of time to get them in, consider the five components of physical fitness: cardiovascular endurance (how high and for how long can you get your heart rate up?), muscular strength (what's the number on those weights?), muscular endurance (how many reps can you do?), flexibility (can you touch your toes?), and body composition (fat versus lean muscle). Taken together, these five components measure total fitness. Kudos to you if you can run a 5K. However, if you can't touch your toes or lift a twenty-pound bag of dog food, then you're not in such good shape after all.

Don't stress—we're not trying to make you feel there's *more* you should be doing. Rather, we want you to think of your fitness holistically and realize these components are interrelated. We want you to turn your frustrations into opportunities. For instance, if you have only ten

MOM 2 MOM

Last winter I took my daughter and a couple of her friends sledding. Something clicked and I was able to see past exercise for alone time, weight maintenance, or race-related goals. I realized I exercise so I can play with my kids and move around in the world with the confidence in my ability to perform physical tasks.

—Kate, mom of two, plus two stepchildren
Indianola, Iowa

minutes to spare, you *can* use that time to advance your fitness. No, you might not be able to get hot and sweaty, but consider where you're falling short among the following five fitness components and use that time to round out your routine.

Broaden Your Definition of Exercise

The following types of exercise each serve a purpose for your overall health and fitness.

1. Therapeutic exercise heals injury or alleviates pain. It maintains a minimal degree of conditioning, say for a woman on bed rest during pregnancy.

2. Protective exercise prevents pain and injury, strengthens weak areas, and keeps the body "in shape" to be in shape.

3. Exercise for physical health meets the minimum exercise requirements—raising your heart rate for thirty minutes most days of the week. It fights heart disease and keeps the number down when we step on the scale.

4. Exercise for mental health gives your brain time to recharge. At the end of a hard day it can mean the difference between tears of joy and tears of frustration.

5. Athletic training challenges the body to meet specific athletic goals. It requires workouts that break us down physically (and sometimes mentally) in order to make us stronger and faster.

Therapeutic Exercise: Yes, That Still Counts

No matter what your age, motherhood strains your body in ways (and places) you previously could not comprehend. Having a baby will provide many "aha" moments, such as: "Aha! That's what Kegel exercises are for." And who knew a three-year-old would still need to be carried (while screaming and flailing his or her arms and legs), or that six-year-olds can run so fast while playing tag?

Therapeutic exercise is called on to treat discomfort or pain. Maybe it's physical therapy for low-back pain, yoga to stretch tight muscles, or a series of strengthening exercises for weak knees.

Sometimes therapeutic exercise is something we do in addition to other workouts; sometimes it's the only alternative. During times of illness, injury, or perhaps a high-risk pregnancy or postpartum period, it's the softer, gentler fitness regimen that replaces more strenuous activity.

What we're saying here is, taking a walk around the neighborhood counts. Stretching for twenty minutes while you play Legos with your son or daughter counts. Calf raises while in line at the grocery store count. Did you break a sweat? Probably not. But strengthening weak or injured areas, stretching tight muscles, or easing up when your body requires it is vital to long-term fitness.

Protective Exercise: An Ounce of Prevention

Protective exercise is the "damage control" from the aging process or playing too hard. For some people this consists of strength training, yoga or Pilates, or an individualized exercise prescription to keep injury-prone areas healthy. Continuing to do these workouts will allow your body to stay injury-free so you are able to do the harder, sweatier stuff.

Like therapeutic exercise, this may or may not be at an intensity that makes you feel you've accomplished any great feat, but it is the core training on which everything else you do is based. Think of protective exercise like a savings account for your body. Making regular, small deposits can accrue interest and "pad" the account, so you can make bigger withdrawals later.

MOM 2 MOM

As a physical therapist I have always been well aware of the need to keep my body balanced and strong. After having my daughter, though, my body was compromised in ways it never was before, and I struggled to feel in shape to even get in shape. I've always looked and felt fit, but picking up a toddler over and over again each day only seemed to enhance my weaknesses, particularly my core. That's when I discovered Pilates. My core has never been stronger and my body remains injury-free. Pilates now encompasses the majority of my workout time, and I realize that not only have I found a new fitness love, but that without it, I couldn't do much else.

—Nancy, mom of one
Dallas, Texas

Exercise for Physical Health: What the Doctor Ordered

You know why you exercise. Your reasons might include the endorphin high, camaraderie from a group workout, skinny jeans, and the thrill of competition. All are fantastic motivators, of course, but the benefits are superfluous, really, compared to saving your life.

Exercise is a major component of chronic disease prevention. Sure, you're thinking, tell me something I don't know. We know you know. We're just reminding you because you might believe that short workouts aren't worth your time. Wrong. Even moderate activity is better than nothing.

If you can't squeeze in an "official workout," you can piece together those efforts you snare throughout your day: park at the far end of the lot, use the stairs instead of the elevator, take jumping-jack breaks while folding laundry, do push-ups while the kids bathe. Some of you may exercise daily without even realizing it. Cleaning house can be exercise, especially when you turn on some tunes and sweep to a beat. Walking your children to the park is a workout (especially if you're pushing seventy pounds of kid in a double stroller). In fact, these are the very kinds of activities the National Institutes of Health, the Centers for Disease Control, and many other health organizations are trying to get the sixty-six million obese people in the United States to do. Five minutes here, ten minutes there, may not seem substantial, but these mini workouts are important.

And for you, when you're in a time or energy crunch, this moderate exercise is what you can hang your sweatband on. Even if your trip to the gym gets cut short and your mind says you didn't work out long enough, chances are your heart and body are still reaping some benefits. In terms of health and longevity, it *is* enough.

MOM 2 MOM

Sometimes all I have time for is a short workout at the gym. Sometimes—especially when I'm traveling—all I do is put on my workout gear and stretch in the hotel fitness center. Even though my life is busy, I can't deny myself a workout several times a week. I know the difference between how my body and mind feel when I'm active and when I'm not, and I owe it to myself and my family to exercise. I do it for the same reasons I prefer organic food, buy nontoxic cleaning products, floss my teeth, and have annual checkups. Simply put, it's good for me.

—Tara, mom of two
Greenbrae, California

Exercise for Mental Health: Save on Therapy

If you were to take an informal poll of fit moms and asked why they exercised, the vast majority would have this to say: stress reduction. Moms stay fit for a number of reasons, but after a hectic day cleaning up mess after mess, convincing children that time really *is* of the essence, trying to get to three different places on time and safely, scrubbing the spot where the toddler peed on the rug again, and finding out the spouse will be home late, getting a workout in has very little to do with dropping a few pounds or trying to prolong your life. (Who needs to live through more days like that?) All you really want to do is breathe.

Remember those Calgon commercials? Isn't the whole idea of getting into a bubble bath to escape the chaos of your day completely unrealistic? In our version of that commercial, kids are banging down the bathroom door, the bathwater is either too hot or too cold, and the trashy novel has fallen into the tub. Relax? Please. Sometimes running away from your problems *is* the answer.

The great part about exercising for mental health is that *any* workout will suffice. If all you have time for is fifteen minutes on the stair-climber, thirty minutes of a yoga tape, a quick spin on the bike, or even a walk around the block, you'll find instant relief from a stressful day.

Athletic Training: Finish Line, Here I Come

When you train, you turn it up a notch both physically and mentally. You push your body and mind beyond your comfort level in hopes of achieving some predetermined goal—whether that's competing at a 5K road race or huffing out a thirty-mile bike ride with a local cycling club. Start training and you stop thinking about exercise as a means of weight

MOM 2 MOM

After my first child was born, I had a serious case of postpartum depression that required I go on medication. I did some research and learned that exercise could help, so I decided to incorporate fitness into my life. Within just a couple of months I was able to eliminate the medication. The more consistent I was, the better I felt and the better my life seemed to be all around. I'm proud that I took control of my health and am setting a good example for my kids. I've gone from being sad and unfit to being fit and happy.

—Melissa, mom of two
Chicago, Illinois

loss or disease prevention. Sure, there's nothing wrong with eliminating those unsightly love handles, it's just that you're more concerned with stepping across the finish line than you are stepping on a scale. The health benefits become secondary to the goals you set for competition.

If you're accustomed to setting (perhaps needing) goals to train by, you know the difficulties you'll face training. You're thinking about performance, which adds direction and purpose to your workouts. It can help you measure success and can even make it easier to justify time spent exercising. Beware of disappointment, though. Who knows what school projects, field trips, or skinned knees will require more time than expected? Being a mom always takes first place, even for the hardcore types. Know yourself. What does it take for you to be happy with your performance? Set yourself up to succeed by setting realistic goals.

In my life before children, I was a regular on the racing scene. Training was a social outlet and I spent most nights and weekends engaged in group workouts and races. My bookshelves were filled with training manuals; my desk overflowed with race entry forms and logbooks. Now that I'm a mom, I've made room for the how-to-raise-your-kid books, and I've definitely cut back on racing. I still train with the same fervor I did before, though, and when I race, I race competitively. Being fit is a huge part of my identity. I train to show my daughters how important and fun it is to live a fit lifestyle. I train because no matter how crazy life gets, a workout makes me feel more grounded. I train to show others it can be done.

—Laurie

Exercise on a Continuum

Exercise that "counts" falls on a continuum from therapeutic to athletic training. As mothers we are faced with many challenges that impact the amount of time and energy we have left for fitness. This dictates where we fall on the exercise continuum at any point in time. It's normal to move from one end of the spectrum to the other—sometimes with little or no warning—on a daily basis. Remember, this is more than just OK; it's actually good for you. Accept, acknowledge, and embrace the variation.

When it comes to taking care of yourself, exercise—regardless of duration or intensity—is the single most important thing you can do. But remember to diversify: Exercise is like eating a balanced diet; you really can have too much of a good thing, especially if you're neglecting certain essentials. You wouldn't just eat from one food group, would you?

Speaking of food, obviously that's an important component of your health, as well. Sometimes finding time for a healthy meal can be as challenging as finding time to work out. It doesn't have to be. Read on.

MOM 2 MOM

After I had my son I started running with a stroller. Soon I was running every day and some days twice a day. After a summer of that I was left with four pelvic stress fractures. That was the best thing that ever happened to me. Because my workouts couldn't include running, I was forced to include strength training and yoga. I branched out and began teaching ballet barre sculpting classes and core fusion in addition to the Pilates that I was already teaching. My diet has evolved and so has my body. And my running has evolved. I'm stronger and faster, but I run only when I feel like running, and I run for fun. I feel balanced on all levels now for the first time in my entire life.

—Michele, mom of one
Minneapolis, Minnesota

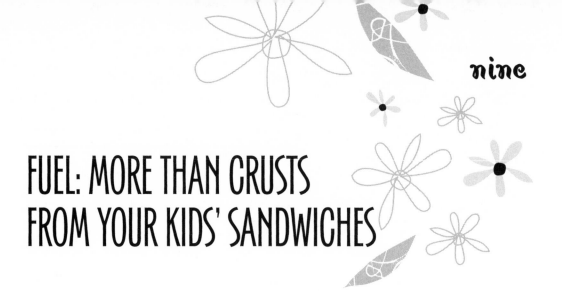

nine

FUEL: MORE THAN CRUSTS FROM YOUR KIDS' SANDWICHES

Our job description as mother often includes food patrol: running interference on our children's food choices, making sure they get enough variety, prodding them to eat their meals so they don't end up snacking later, and, of course, preventing vegetables from "falling off the table" into the dog's mouth.

We want to make sure our kids properly fuel their bodies, but do we approach our own nutrition with the same vigilance? Mothers simply can't overlook their own good nutrition, especially if making it through a workout is part of their day. But what should we be eating? And when? And if you're trying to feed, clothe, and raise children, too, then *how*?

Check out your local bookstore and you'll see as many opinions on food consumption as theories for raising your children. But even when you know how to eat right, putting those good habits to practice is the hard part. It's not just *what* you eat that helps fuel your fitness, it's also *when*, *how*, and *why*.

What We Eat—Cross-Training for Your Diet

You may already subscribe to certain nutrition principles, or maybe you've adopted a particular way of eating made famous by a diet guru or nutrition expert. Maybe your preference for roasted sweet potatoes over French fries comes naturally. If you already make healthy eating coexist with your fit life, congratulations! Good nutrition and physical activity belong together, and together they will give your life some crazy good synergy.

However, if healthy food is your nemesis and you tend to get overwhelmed with all the "advice" about good nutrition, we have an approach for you that's simple out of necessity for busy moms like us.

Eating healthy shouldn't be complicated. But you've said that about getting new toys out of those horrific plastic clamshell packages, right? We mean it. In fact, it's so simple that it's part of elementary education. Yup, we're talking about the food pyramid. There are just six things to remember—things we know you've heard, perhaps have already adopted. We've just added our own fit-mom twist:

Load up on veggies. All of that oxygen you use during a workout creates free radicals in your body, which have been known to cause everything from wrinkles to cancer. The antioxidant vitamins found in vegetables neutralize free radicals, so aim for fresh or frozen, which hold on to their nutrients better. If you eat ten servings of vegetables a day and are still hungry for dessert, then go for it!

Fixate on fruit. Fruit is packed with antioxidants just like your veggies. Opt to keep the skin on fruits such as apples and pears to benefit from the fiber. Think whole. But don't be fooled by fruit juices. Juices are packed with excess sugar, and too much juice contributes to obesity, cavities, diarrhea, gas, and bloating—none of which make for comfortable workouts.

Go lean on protein. Active moms, especially, can't skimp on protein. It's what builds and repairs those muscles after you give them a good whopping. Feed your muscles wisely, though. Skip the fried chicken. And think beyond meat and fish to beans, legumes, nuts, and seeds. In a pinch you can turn to protein bars, but check out the ingredients and make sure they're not glorified candy bars.

Eat calcium-rich foods. Women who work out have a higher need for calcium than their sedentary friends. Stress fractures are a real worry, especially for women who run, walk, or do other weight-bearing activities. If you love dairy, this might be easy. Rather than nonfat, choose dairy with a little fat, which has been shown to be the vehicle that carries dairy's nutrients; in other words, fat-soluble vitamins may not "stick to your ribs" without it. Some cereals and juices come fortified with calcium; just don't forget about those sneaky sugars. Other foods can provide a calcium boost, too: broccoli, dark leafy greens, salmon, and tofu.

Eat whole grains. Don't give up on bread and pasta just yet. Because carbohydrates are easily converted to energy, they fuel our fitness. Without them, you'll feel fatigued. The changeup here is to choose "whole" over "enriched" grains and seek out grains as close to their natural state as possible. Whole grains aren't just rich in fiber (we all know how fiber helps us start the day right); they are full of vitamins and minerals, too. Be mindful of portion sizes, however. Discovering the real serving for a bowl of cereal, for instance, can be sobering.

Include healthy fats. The good news is you *do* need fat in your diet. Everyone does. You need those essential fatty acids in order to keep your immune system strong. And for a fit mom, strong immunity equals strong body. With kids in the house, you're constantly dodging illness. Good fat keeps your force field up. The challenge is to become proficient in detecting good versus bad fat, because the bad fats don't boost your immunity; oftentimes they do just the opposite. Steer away from solid fats, such as those in shortening or lard. Cook with unsaturated fats in plant foods and opt for oils and foods such as salmon, walnuts, and flax that boost your intake of essential fatty acids.

Healthy eating really is that simple—simpler, too, if you're good at limiting your sweets and salts (and alcohol, too, while we're mentioning moderation). Lastly, pay attention to portion sizes (packaged goods are typically more than one serving) and be aware of (but not obsessive about!) the number of calories you consume in a day.

Whatever you're eating should be appropriate for the whole family and vice versa. Why should it be any different? Remember, you're not a short-order cook. Kids will see you eat well and mimic that behavior, and then, we hope, go on to establish a lifelong pattern of healthy nutrition. For example, if you want your children to eat their fruits and vegetables, it's best you dig into those Brussels sprouts yourself. You may not love the taste, but your body loves what they provide in terms of nutrients and fiber. Try to get your taste buds (or theirs) to come around by preparing the "yucky" vegetables in a new way. Explore your options and try one new vegetable each month. Hit your local farmers' market on the weekends—you'll be surprised by how many are available and in season.

Likewise, make sure your rules limiting sweets and sodas apply not just to your kids, but to you as well. Are your kids limited to two or three cookies? Then limit yourself, too. That means you shouldn't finish the entire package

> Someday my children are going to catch me eating an extra cookie and call out my hypocrisy. I justify my higher cookie count in various ways: chief among them that while they don't need the sugar buzz, I do!
>
> —Kara

after they go to bed. Eliminating hypocrisy from your diet will make you feel good as well as help you control your sweet tooth.

When We Eat—Intentional Ingestion

Whatever happened to breakfast, lunch, and dinner? "Three squares" might be the convention for our children, but not for moms who are working their waitress shift: cooking, serving, getting up for a glass of milk, up again for a spoon, up again for another napkin, up again to refill the milk. By the time you sit down long enough to get in three bites of food, everyone has left the table and it's time to clear the dirty dishes. Why bother?

Well, as futile as it may seem, those three meals are the anchors to your caloric needs. Especially breakfast. Sure, you could consume the total amount of calories you need to sustain your day in one sitting, but our tanks are not designed to be "filled up" like cars. We exert energy throughout the day and likewise we need to take in energy as needed—and even to stay one step ahead of our energy expenditures.

Sometimes, though, it's easier on us mentally if we feed the kids first and nibble throughout the day. Even if you succeed in accumulating enough bites to equal a balanced meal, you might miss the mark nutritionally by under- or overestimating your needs.

Although we're not endorsing mindless grazing, we believe snack food has its place; crackers, fruit, and sandwich crusts work great to keep hunger at bay during your busy day. (Admit it, PB&J crusts aren't so bad!) But snacking *all* day won't sustain both mom *and* athlete.

Small, intentional meals combined with healthy snacks work best. Keep it real—real food, that is. Ask yourself if what you're about to pop in your mouth will power your workout. If you've ever felt the difference in how your body performs on candy versus healthy food, making that choice is much easier.

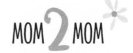

And speaking of working out, don't get caught with an empty stomach or, worse, with a too-full stomach just before you engage in exercise. Every digestive system has its own unique requirements for what it will tolerate and when in relation to exercise, so experiment with easy-to-digest foods and their proximity to your workout (this may be different depending on the intensity). Refer back to chapter 7, "Fitness SOS," where we answer the question "Should I eat now or wait until *after* my workout?"

How We Eat—Sit Down, Slow Down, and Savor

As described above, busy moms usually find themselves eating their meals as they cook, serve, and attend to their families at mealtime. This is no way to eat. As hard as it may be, try to sit down to eat your meals. Call for a twenty-minute moratorium on second helpings; that's how long it takes your brain to register that you've eaten enough.

MOM 2 MOM

Once a week we have a giant snack night (my husband invented it). I put out healthy foods in small dishes and everyone can pick and choose what they prefer.

—Kathy, mom of two
Kansas City, Kansas

Develop some dining room traditions that require everyone's presence. Go around the table for a quick game of "best and worst" (moments of the day, that is; don't ask your kids' opinion about what's on their plate). Take turns coming up with a "question of the day." Don't call anyone to the table until everything is ready lest the food get eaten before you take a seat. When your kids are old enough, expect some independence: Let them get their own spoon when that fork you provided just won't do. Do whatever else you can to prevent getting up. One idea is to put dinner on the table allowing everyone to help themselves (build your own tacos, sandwiches, or salads). If kids "make it" themselves, they are more likely to eat it. And by all means enable children to retrieve those extra napkins or refill their own cups of milk.

Sitting down to eat meals does this: First and foremost it allows us to eat mindfully. For once, we suggest, *do not multitask*. Just sit and eat. Chew your food well and you're more likely to enjoy it and feel satiated. Pay attention to what goes in and when you feel full. And when you feel full? Yes, that's right, *stop eating*.

We realize this kind of meal is ideal but not always possible. As we mentioned above, active moms on the go may find themselves eating

As a nibbler who is typically done with a meal before it even hits the table, I know I eat less if I wait and enjoy the final product (but that doesn't apply to cookie dough).

—Laurie

on the run. When you do, be prepared. It's better to take in foods that are quickly digested without the refined sugar—banana, yogurt, nuts, dried fruit. If you're always on the move, pack healthy snacks in your bag or keep them in your desk and car. Make it easier to eat healthy than eat junk food.

Why We Eat—Hunger or Food Therapy?

What makes us eat? Ideally hunger, right? If you're eating for the right reasons, you're eating to fuel your body for fitness, which in turn fuels your lifestyle.

Sometimes, though, it's anxiety that fuels our appetite. Eating can become a weapon to combat boredom, a drug to fight depression. There's a good reason certain foods are called "comfort foods." Eating carbohydrates boosts serotonin levels—the "happy hormone" that really can make us feel better. The problem, of course, is they can also make us fatter. But you, enlightened active mama, know what else raises serotonin. That's right: exercise.

If you're in need of a serotonin boost, of course, we suggest trying exercise first. But sometimes we need to succumb to our cravings. And you know what? That's OK. But set up some ground rules first. Set realistic limits. You might consider making yourself eat a carrot stick or an apple before you scarf that cupcake. (What's the fun in that? None, really, but at least you'll get some nutritive value from a fruit or veggie along with the sugar surge.) Or, if you indulge and then find yourself clamoring for more, step away. Get up and do something else. Make a deal that you can't have a second helping for twenty minutes. You still want it? Bets are you will. In either case you're not denying yourself—just delaying gratification. Hopefully, you won't be hungry after those twenty minutes have passed.

Another good idea is to have "acceptable indulgences" available—perhaps sugar-free fudgesicles, low-fat ice cream, or your own low-fat, low-sugar concoction of choice. Find a dessert you can still feel good about. It's not a bad idea to treat yourself; just be discerning when it comes to the treats you choose.

If you find emotional eating gets the best of you, then you may have more work to do than setting up boundaries. If your caloric consumption is directly proportional to how much stress you feel in life, start paying attention to your food triggers. You might need

> I hear vegan black bean brownies are delicious. If you've tried them and concur, I'll believe you.
>
> —Kara

professional help to break the cycle of feeding your stress. Likewise, if stress turns off your taste buds or you battle with an eating disorder, seek professional help.

Ensure Your Energy

Enough of the right kind of food should adequately cover our energy expenditures. *Should*. But when you heap on more exercise, more birthdays, and more stress, sometimes we fall short. Even though we believe strongly in the perking-up power of coffee, it's important to take out some insurance for your "recommended daily allowance" of vitamins and minerals.

Yes, whole food choices are better because they pack a nutritional punch that a supplement can't deliver. For instance, a strawberry isn't just a dose of vitamin C. Yes, one serving of fresh strawberries contributes 140 percent of the recommended daily value of vitamin C, but it also packs in 20 percent of folic acid needs, some potassium, fiber, and the phytochemicals that protect against a host of chronic illnesses such as cancer, heart disease, and diabetes. No vitamin C supplement can do all that.

But there will be those days when all you *do* get are the crusts from your kids' sandwiches. On those "off days" when you're stretching to reach the peak of the food pyramid (Does ketchup count as a vegetable?) be sure to take vitamins and other nutritional supplements that give your day some oomph. As much as we try to do right by giving our body sleep and healthy food, we can't help the gaps.

For most pregnant and lactating moms, taking a prenatal vitamin is routine. Then, years pass and we find ourselves popping a few gummy bear vitamins while we dole them out to our kids. Find a multi that provides 100 percent of the recommended daily value for most vitamins and minerals, and take it. In addition, the most important letters on the bottle aren't necessarily A, B, or C; they're USP, which stand for United States Pharmacopeia. This indicates the brand meets formulation standards.

In addition to filling in the gaps with a good multivitamin, meeting (and in some cases, exceeding) those daily values can play a pivotal role in women's wellness and disease prevention.

While most multivitamins will help you reach the recommended daily value established by the U.S. Food and Drug Administration (see box below) you might talk with your health care provider or nutritionist about whether your needs exceed those recommendations (so long as they don't surpass the upper level intake established, which could be toxic and cause side effects).

Are You Getting Enough of These Nutrients?

	Women under 50	Women over 50	What's it do?
Calcium	1,000 milligrams	1,200 milligrams	Keeps bones strong
Vitamin D	5 micrograms	10 micrograms	Helps with calcium absorption; helps prevent a host of illnesses; minimizes PMS
Magnesium	310 milligrams (under 30)	320 milligrams (over 30)	Helps with calcium absorption
Folic Acid	400 micrograms	400 micrograms	Prevents birth defects; keeps your heart healthy
B_6	1.3 milligrams	1.5 milligrams	Keeps your heart healthy; combats stress
B_{12}	2.4 micrograms	2.4 micrograms	Keeps your heart healthy; combats stress

Moms who exceed moderate exercise should consider supplementation, too. Talk to your doctor about extra antioxidants, especially vitamins C, E, and selenium, which are helpful in repairing damaged cells. Other supplements that may prove useful for fit moms include:

Essential Fatty Acids (Omega 3, 6, and 9): Our bodies can't make essential fatty acids, or EFAs, on their own, so without eating foods rich in these (think salmon, flax, and walnuts) or supplements, we would miss out on their benefits, including improved heart health, anti-inflammatory properties, and a boost to brain power. If you're pregnant or nursing these are especially important to a developing neurological system.

Glucosamine/Chondroitin: Some studies show how these two supplements work together to improve joint pain. The study participants had arthritis, but athletes who have put their knees and/or hips through too many miles might reap the same benefits. Try the supplement for three months. If you feel improvement, it may be worth the money.

Probiotics: No one wants their body overrun by too much "bad" bacteria, which can cause tummy trouble, intestinal distress, and the dreaded yeast infection. It's like your home—the more security you have, the less inviting it is for the bad guys. You can invest in this "security system" for your immune system by eating yogurt and drinking kefir (and you'll boost your calcium while you're at it). You can also supplement with probiotic capsules—find them in the refrigerated section at your health food store.

Super antioxidants: Certain foods are far superior in delivering antioxidant benefits to our bodies—foods such as berries, kiwi, and the latest superfood de jour: the chia seed (not just for chia pets anymore). Some companies offer supplemental versions that allow you all the potency in a small serving, tablet, or bar, versus consuming an entire crate of produce.

All the above supplements *may* help add to your energy stores—and in some cases have proven benefits—but there isn't one answer for everyone. You may find that particular foods or certain vitamins and supplements give you a noticeable boost; others, not so much. But even if you don't perk up to the extent you hope, at least you'll lower your risk for cancer, osteoporosis, and heart disease, among other things. And if these vitamins, minerals, and supplements can do all that, then it's possible they can put an extra spring in your step, too. We're all for help creating energy—even if it's the placebo effect.

Kitchen Makeover

Marble countertops and stainless steel appliances might make for a dream kitchen. But as a fit mom your dream of convenient, healthy meals takes more than a good contractor. What's important is stocking your kitchen with healthy food and helpful equipment that keeps you moving in high gear all day long.

Ingredients for a Healthy Kitchen

It's time to take inventory in your kitchen. What are your dietary staples? Take some time to look over the nutritional information more closely. Are there changes you can make to your everyday foods that will add a little gusto to your day? Eliminate foods that are lacking in nutritional content and replace them with healthy alternatives.

Toss

- White enriched grain products, such as rice and bread.
- Any product with hydrogenated oil of any kind.
- Packaged products that list sugar in the top three ingredients (check your cereal labels).
- Products containing high fructose corn syrup (check labels on fruit juices).

Buy

- Whole grains, such as oatmeal, brown rice, quinoa, millet, and barley.
- At least three varieties of fresh vegetables and three varieties of fresh fruit each week. Consider a share from a farm with a Community-Supported Agriculture (CSA) program. You'll get a weekly supply of vegetables, and sometimes fruit, that are at their seasonal peak, locally grown, and often organic.
- Fish, for meals at least twice a week.

Replace

- Yogurt juice with kefir.
- Vegetable oil with ground flax seed (3 tablespoons of flax seed for every 1 tablespoon of vegetable oil when baking).
- Traditional margarine with nonhydrogenated spreads.
- Peanut oil with olive, walnut, or canola oil.
- One meat meal a week with a vegetarian meal featuring lentils or beans.

Become a "Gear Geek"

Exercise accessories and gadgets make it easier for you to meet your fitness goals by offering convenience, accessibility, and insight. Same concept applies in the kitchen. Here are some smart buys for that fit-mom dream kitchen:

- **Blender** for smoothies and soups. Toss in some fruit, yogurt, and a little ice and you've got a healthy treat.
- **Steamer** for vegetables and brown rice. These babies cook to tender perfection, making veggies tastier, even for the kids.
- **Countertop grill** for cooking poultry and fish quickly. This is a great way to fit in protein without the hassle and puts a little sizzle into sandwich night.

- **Atomizer** for oil. Cooking with olive oil is good for you, and you can avoid overdoing it by spraying it on instead of pouring it on.
- **Slow cooker** for no-stress meals. Toss in your favorite meat and veggies before you leave in the morning and your meal is ready when you get home.

Tips and Techniques for Efficient Food Prep

You've got the food, you've got the means to cook. Still not easy, right? It's all about convenience. Let's face it, it's much easier to grab a handful of chips or a pack of Pop-Tarts and head out the door than it is to peel and cut some healthy veggies. Here are our best bets for making healthy eating more convenient:

- Wash, cut, and store vegetables so they're easily accessible and ready to eat. Take care of this "burden" as soon as possible after returning from the grocery store or you'll end up with good intentions and spoiled veggies.
- Keep a bowl of fresh fruit on the counter, table, or in some other visible location. Like those veggies, get them washed ahead of time and rid yourself of one less barrier to eating right.
- Make your own snack cups in the form of "individual servings," using (and reusing) zip-top bags or plastic containers that you can take on the go.
- Silence the taunts of your "temptation foods" by keeping them out of the house altogether. If that isn't possible, stash those goodies out of reach—perhaps in a cupboard that requires a stepstool or a few extra steps.
- Let slow-cooking grains soak during the day (for dinner) or overnight (for breakfast) and cut cooking time in half.
- If, like your two-year-old, you find yourself feeding certain veggies to the dog, don't give up. Find three recipes that incorporate the food before giving up on it entirely. You're likely to find an appealing concoction. And who knows, your two-year-old might even like it, too.
- Double up whenever you can and freeze the extras. On the weekend when you have time to make pancakes, freeze leftovers for quick, toaster-oven ready cakes. Make extra soup or pasta and freeze it for emergency meals.

■ Do your homework and find a few "best bet" recipes. These are healthy alternatives you know everyone will eat willingly. Make these recipes staples in your weekly menu planning.

Get yourself eating right and you'll find that you have more energy for taking on life as a fit mom. Heck, it might be the difference between walking around like a zombie and actually noticing those flowers you don't have time to smell. However, eating right isn't enough. You have to give your body time to recover, your battery time to recharge. More on that in the next chapter.

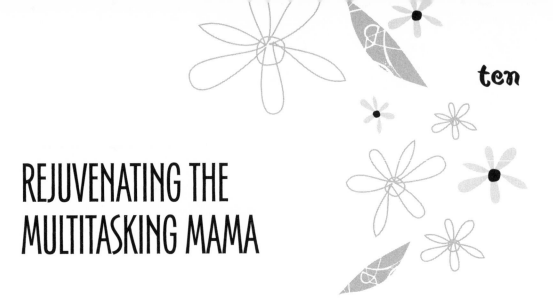

ten

REJUVENATING THE MULTITASKING MAMA

Let's face it: When someone asks you if you're "getting enough," you assume they're talking about sleep. It's not that you've lost your libido, it's just that sleep—rock-hard, solid sleep—is what you really lust for. Dim the lights, climb under the covers, and get your eight hours. Now *that's* sexy.

Odds are you're not too tired just for sex. You're probably too tired for a lot of other things—taking on that massive grocery run, cleaning off the mixture of crackers and juice that is now plastered inside your car, and the forty-five-minute workout you wanted to get in today. Really, how can you expect to have sex when you fall asleep just a half page into that novel you've been trying to read for the last year?

You're not just tired. You're exhausted. It's time to rejuvenate.

Re · ju · ve · nate \ri-'jü-və-nāt\: 1. To make young again; restore to youthful vigor or appearance. 2. To restore to a former state; make fresh or new again.

How do you make yourself "fresh or new again"? It's not as simple as wolfing down an energy bar or taking a quick power nap. No, when you're really exhausted, as in I-could-sleep-for-two-days-straight-and-still-be-tired exhausted, you've got to sip energy from everything and anything out there, not just your favorite coffee mug.

Rest

Rest \'rest\: The most obvious antidote for a tired, crabby mom. Created by spending hours in pajamas in the absence of children, shirking responsibilities, and indulging in leisure.

You know when your kids need a nap, right? They get overemotional, whiny, clingy. The first sign of this behavior and you're likely to abandon the grocery cart, ask for a to-go container, or cut that playdate short. Usually the loose cannon is back under control after a nap or some "alone time."

Sleep deprivation also has debilitating effects for grown-ups, including compromised immunity and physical performance (at the gym *or* in bed). It can impair your mind, too. Obvious signs you need more sleep include squeezing the tube of Bengay, instead of toothpaste, on your toothbrush; starting a pot of coffee without first putting coffee in the filter; finding your lost sunglasses on top of your head. And, yes, you might also find yourself overemotional, whiny, and clingy.

Rest is the perfect remedy for a crabby kid. So what about a tired, crabby mom? Here are a few tactics for squeezing some rest into your (yes, we know) already busy day.

Take a Timeout

Taking a timeout or engaging in some quiet time might seem like a luxury, rather than a necessity. But, if you really want to feel energetic and get your game face back, it's probably the best medicine out there. Employers are required to provide breaks; demand no less for yourself, even if you work at home. Take a few deep breaths, read a favorite inspiring passage, or just close your eyes and escape to your favorite place (whether you've been there or not).

At home, establish a "take a break" chair or timeout location that can be used by everyone in the family. If you've been behaving badly and give yourself a timeout, your children will have

> I like to coordinate mindless laundry folding with some afternoon television. When the kids come in while I'm watching Oprah and see I'm folding laundry they immediately turn around and leave. They want no part of laundry folding. Then I can shove the pile of clothes on the floor and put my feet up for a few minutes. As far as the kids know, I'm folding laundry.
>
> —Kara

all the more respect for you. Give them the option for voluntary breaks, too. Show your children that it's OK to withdraw for a few minutes to inhale a few breaths of sanity. And remember to respect one another's privacy during a self-induced break. Everyone in the family should honor the boundary for this retreat within your home.

Set Your Alarm (Morning and Night)

Perhaps those days of actually needing an alarm clock are long gone. Even mothers of teenagers will tell you they rarely sleep through the night. We know we need more sleep and long for those rare mornings when we can sleep in. Even so, don't throw away your alarm clock altogether. You may need to use it to remind yourself what time to go to sleep. Sleep experts advise going to bed and waking up at the same time each day and allowing for at least seven hours of sleep each night (eight is preferable, but we're being realistic).

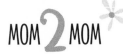

MOM 2 MOM

If I sleep through my alarm, it probably means I needed sleep more than a workout.

—Sara, mom of one
Minneapolis, Minnesota

Maintaining a strict sleep schedule takes discipline, especially if you're a night owl and don't have the extra time in the morning (due to a child who is an early riser, a school schedule, or a work schedule). If you're a fan of the late-night shows, seriously consider a digital video recorder. No one says you have to watch the late-night shows late at night. If you're staying up late to work or clean the house, ask yourself if compromising sleep to get that work done is really necessary. Yes, sometimes in order to meet certain obligations (or visiting in-laws) we do need to work a little overtime. Just don't make a habit out of it. Skimping on sleep should be in the same category as indulging in your favorite gooey dessert: things to do sparingly.

Develop a Sleep Ritual

If you have trouble shutting down at night, create a sleep ritual. This is the same sound advice we use when helping our babies reset their biological clocks away from daytime sleep toward more nighttime sleep. Even as adults, our biological clocks use recurring cues to signal our sympathetic nervous system to begin certain actions, such as secrete the sleep hormone melatonin. That's why getting up and going to bed at the same time is so helpful. If you're struggling with the going-to-bed part, pick certain things to do, just before bed, to signal your body that now is the time to shut down. Perhaps drink chamomile tea, read, and slather lavender lotion on your hands and feet. Maybe the ten o'clock news, writing in a journal, or working on a crossword puzzle is your cue. It doesn't matter what you do (although do try to make the activity calming) so long as you provide your body with recurring signals (taste, smell, actions) that indicate sleep will be next.

If you are having trouble shutting down, then regular exercise has another benefit for you. Research shows that exercise is as effective as other options for treating insomnia. Experiment with different intensities and times of day, and try to exercise outdoors for the added benefit of light exposure, which helps synchronize your biological clock and gives you a dose of vitamin D, a natural antidepressant. Just a reminder ladies: this sleep aid isn't a pill, it's *exercise*.

Create Your Own Sleep Sanctuary

Another way to honor your need for sleep is to make your bed and bedroom a sleep sanctuary. Other than sex, everything else you do there should be designed to induce sleep. (Even if you think you're too tired for sex, there's nothing like a good orgasm to put you to sleep.)

Give sleep the reverence it deserves by making your bedroom a shrine for sleep. Paint a sleep-inducing color on the walls and put up dark shades or black-out curtains to minimize light. Invest in (or scour the sale bins for) quality sheets and pillows. We'd like to add white noise or earplugs to block out sound, but we understand that hearing a young child in distress is part of duty calling. On that note, however, do rethink your baby monitor, if you're still using one. If your child is in the room next to you, do you need to hear every gurgle, snort, and fart? If your kid really needs you, we all know they're loud enough to get us in that room, no monitor required.

Speaking of baby paraphernalia, what else can you boot from your room? Legos between the sheets will surely sabotage your sleep. Keep toys out of your room and minimize your own clutter. Stacks and piles of any sort can represent the stress that's keeping us from sleep.

If you're already conditioned to poor sleep because you worry about it and associate your bedroom with wake-filled nights, simply going to bed in a different room for one or two nights might help you sleep better.

Teach Your Kids to Sleep

Good sleep habits beget good sleep habits. If your children are getting adequate sleep (and we're not about to tell you how to do *that*) then you have better odds of adequate sleep, too. So, try to establish a regular sleep routine for your children and be persistent in the early years. It will pay off down the road.

Whenever my husband and I had particularly grueling bouts with waking kids (newborn twins, anyone?), we took turns sleeping in the basement in order to get a full night of shut-eye. Even one good night's sleep can reverse the trend of sleep anxiety that we'd feel, worrying when the next kid would wake us up.

—Kara

Sleep Appraisal

There are two types of tired: "sleepy" and "fatigued." Sleepy is what you might experience during that midafternoon slump or the lull you get on the drive home from work. Do you want to work out? No. Should you work out? Yes.

Fatigue is a whole different conundrum. Fatigue is being washed over with inertia, down to your core, so that the act of getting out of bed becomes an "event," and getting in the shower, a finish line of sorts. Fatigue requires you to back off. But being sleepy, well, you need to kick it in the pants.

The "take time, make time, share time, and snare time" method of finding a way to work out applies to getting a nap, too. If you've reached the point of exhaustion, supplementing sleep with a nap helps you survive, literally. Driving while sleep deprived is similar to driving while intoxicated. Getting less than six hours of sleep triples your risk of getting into a car accident. In addition, less than six hours of shut-eye increases your odds of picking up a viral infection by

MOM 2 MOM

My second daughter was not a good sleeper. I was up throughout the night during her first year. I was exhausted, but I wanted to run, and after shoving myself into those too-tight sports bras and running four miles, I got mastitis. I just didn't have the reserves. I reached a point where I should have taken a nap instead of gone running.

—Kate, mom of two
Minneapolis, Minnesota

50 percent. The chances of having a heart attack and stroke are also higher in people who skimp on sleep. When we say "survive," we mean it.

If you're getting less than seven hours of sleep at night, a power nap is a better pick-me-up than a caffeine-spiked drink. Most people experience a lull about eight hours after waking. Research shows that a little midday sleep can improve brain function, reduce stress, and increase efficiency for the remainder of the day. So, when you head into those early evening "witching hours," you, at least, will not be a witch.

Even though you may feel as if you could nap for hours, you don't need to. Experts recommend somewhere between fifteen and thirty minutes. Studies show that twenty minutes of afternoon sleep is more beneficial to the body than twenty minutes of extra sleep in the morning.

If you think a nap is frivolous, remind yourself of the restorative powers of sleep. What's a nap (and its benefits) worth to you?

Cross-Training

cross-train \krôs'-trān'\: Adding variety to your fitness regimen by moving your body in new ways; stepping outside the ordinary to rev up your enthusiasm for working out.

When you're sleepy and not motivated to work out, you don't want to do the Same. Old. Thing. Cross-training can help you break out of a rut and turn that midafternoon slump or postwork lull into exercise foreplay. The promise of excitement, newness, sizzle: It's like dating someone for the first time.

If you've been exercising for any length of time, you've probably discovered the joys of cross-training. Alternating the type of workout, say from running to swimming, or adding extra time in another discipline, helps prevent and heal overuse injuries as well as develop muscular balance. That's all well and good, but it can't hold a candle to sizzle.

So here's what you may need (especially if you're already familiar with cross-training— even your cross-training may be ho-hum). Go beyond cross-training; go beyond what's familiar. Who cares if you're good at it? Not only will you challenge your body, but you'll also engage your brain to learn new skills. Go rock climbing, dust off your roller blades, and—our personal favorite—take a hip-hop class.

In order for this "blind-date exercise" to work for you, you must have an open mind. Don't pooh-pooh that kickboxing class because you lack rhythm. Don't think that group cycling class is out of your league. Don't roll your eyes at the buff boot-camp instructor. Don't bypass the pool because, well, just because. When you're feeling stale, unmotivated, or just too tired to get that workout in, it's time for sizzle. Allowing for a little sizzle in your fitness plan can prevent you from complete burnout.

Immunity

Immunity \i-'myü-nə-tē\: Your first line of defense for staying in the game, on the bike, or on the trails. Typically acquired after exposure from a virus, but best obtained through more protective measures.

If you get sick you'll need more than rejuvenation; you'll need a full body overhaul. So kiss your kids at your own risk. You are not just mother to your children, you are also mother to the germs they host and as such, you often become host to them, too.

But we adore our contagious little angels who rob us of our immune systems while filling us with love. So short of wearing a gas mask, the best way to avoid a viral or bacterial infestation is to wash your hands. Obsessively. Of course, you do this after you use the restroom, but scrub up anytime you've been out in public, too—especially the gym, which can play host to a multitude of nasty germs. And definitely carry antibacterial wipes and sanitizer for a quick wipe down of the shopping cart, tabletop, and other germ-infested surfaces. Short of becoming agoraphobic, consider limiting outings to high-traffic kid places when you really can't afford the time or energy to be sick. Don't even go near any of those fast-food indoor playgrounds, unless you *want* a side of stomach flu with that kids' meal.

Exercise, once again, can play a role here, too. If you exercise moderately and consistently, on a near-daily basis, you can increase the circulation of immune cells that kill off viruses and bacteria. After exercise ends, this heightened immune function

MOM 2 MOM

Before, if I felt even slightly tired or a little cold coming on, I'd skip my workout. Now, I'm to the point where I feel worse if I skip it, than if I'd gone.

—Sara, mom of two
Walla Walla, Washington

returns to normal, but if you keep up with the exercise regularly you provide your body with a natural, daily immunization. Again: not a pill, just a little exercise. Amazing, isn't it?

Despite whatever arsenal you use to ward off germs, if you feel something coming on—don't be caught off guard. Coddle your immune system with vigilant nutrition, and back off on exercise as necessary in order to sneak in extra rest to give your body the energy required to fight the illness. Finally, hold fast to the thought that if you are healthy, you'll only get a mild version of what everyone else has. (This may be difficult while hugging the toilet, but a little optimism can't hurt.)

Mama Zen

Mama Zen /ma-ma/ /'zen/: Getting in touch with that poised, calm, and controlled woman inside by connecting mind, body, and soul.

Taking your mind, body, and spirit to a different level is, truly, one more thing to do. Building a sense of calm may take effort, but like exercise, the benefits pay off and are palpable. Once you've been exposed to a sense of peace, even a teeny tiny bit of inner peace, you'll know it's there for you to access, to grab on to when you need it. Also, once you know that that calm, peaceful woman resides inside you, you become better at channeling her and acquiring that peace on demand (and for longer periods). Like exercise, once you feel the benefits you'll crave more. There's no recipe or road map to inner peace. However, there are a few tried and true methods. We are not, after all, the first humans on the planet after a little Zen.

Meditate

As you read this book, take note of your body. Is your brow furrowed? Are the corners of your mouth pursed and your jaw clenched? Are your shoulders creeping up toward your ears?

Now take a minute to relax and just breathe. Listen to yourself inhale and exhale, paying attention to nothing but the sound and feel of your breath, and let go. When thoughts cloud

> The last time I tried to get a little alone time on the potty, my youngest barged in on me three times in less than five minutes. My desperation was muted by her final plea to stay: "I'll wipe you."
>
> —Laurie

your mind, label them (planning, anxiety, and so on), accept them for what they are without judgment, and watch them float away. Then adjust your thinking to do nothing but focus on the breath.

That's meditation in a nutshell—an age-old way of reducing anxiety and stress. You're not looking for a big epiphany. No nudging yourself closer to Nirvana. No need to search for Nirvana. Heck, you don't even need to know what Nirvana is. It's about living in the present moment and accepting where you are—adapting that recognition of breath to everyday life. Get this down and a toddler tantrum becomes bearable.

If you must, lock yourself in the bathroom (tell them you're going number two, even if you're not) or sit in your car an extra minute after taking the kids to school or yourself to work; find a few moments each day to simply breathe. Even if all you do is take three deep breaths, you'll be amazed by how much stress you unleash and energy you capture. If a power nap isn't for you, a few minutes of meditation will provide the same benefits. You can even make this a "moving meditation" on your next walk or run.

> The benefits of a few deep breaths help my kids deal with stress. Sometimes the only way to diffuse the drama is to hold their hands while they slowly inhale and exhale.
>
> —Kara

Yoga and Tai Chi

You can also clear your mind while working the stress and kinks out of your body. Many great practices such as yoga and tai chi provide excellent mind-body workouts. Go ahead, give something new a try.

Don't be intimidated by those limber yogis. The wonderful thing about yoga is that it offers something for everyone—from basic moves such as downward-facing dog and child's pose, both restorative and restful in nature, to more challenging poses such as headstand and balancing half-moon that test your balance and put some zing into your circulation.

Originating in India, yoga has been around for more than five thousand years. The physical practice of yoga that Westerners are familiar

> Don't get too caught up in your breath when you start a yoga practice. As a beginner, I fell flat on my face once doing that. As luck would have it, the studio was packed. Relax. In no time, proper breathing will become second nature.
>
> —Laurie

with is just one component of a traditional yoga practice and was created in part to offer relief for monks who sat in meditation for hours on end. These ancient postures still have applications for counteracting our modern-day bad habits that perpetuate poor alignment and tense muscles (most notably, sitting too much). Yoga also integrates breath with all of the postures so you become more in tune to how breathing affects your body.

Another popular mind-body practice is tai chi, which originated in China and is often described as meditation in motion. Tai chi consists of a series of flowing movements that focus on balance, strength, and agility while incorporating a focus on breath. Tai chi is done while standing and taking steps. Your legs provide a strong foundation while you move your arms slowly and purposefully through the air.

Whether you choose to make a yoga or tai chi class a regular stop on your schedule or adopt a few poses or sequences you can do at home on your own, developing a regular practice not only creates suppleness in your limbs but promotes mindfulness as well. We like those kind of twofer deals.

Spirit

If you are (or want to be) a spiritual person, don't forget to train this aspect of your life, too. There is an amazing connection between our spiritual selves and our physical selves beyond providing motivation (no, you won't go to hell if you skip worship for a workout!). Regardless of your spiritual beliefs, taking time to access strength from a higher power (or wherever you get your mojo) will boost your energy level and help center your soul. How much time you need to focus on this aspect of your life is completely personal. Figure out what your spirit craves and fill up. Some of us get everything we need from a weekly visit to our church, synagogue, or mosque. For others, getting involved in a charity or volunteering at a local food shelter may be what sustains their spirit. By all means pray while out on a walk or run. Sometimes the simple act of moving your body and recognizing that you are alive instigates a spontaneous outpouring of gratitude. So while you're celebrating your body, say "thank you" to whomever you feel it is owed.

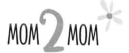

I exercise to honor God for my good health. The least I can do is honor His temple (my body) and take good care of it.

—Joanna, mom of two
San Antonio, Texas

Pamper

Pamper \pam-pər\: To care for with indulgence. Something moms naturally do for others but rarely enjoy themselves.

The diaper folks got it right. What mom doesn't want to pamper her child? We're not endorsing any brands here, but the name says it all. We don't expect you to cram into your toddler's diaper, but you can pamper yourself with whatever makes you feel good. And if you haven't figured it out by now, it's OK to feel good. Having the confidence to be pampered is part of the luxury. Surely we've already established that you're a worthwhile, deserving member of the family who can step up and voice her needs. Every single one of us has a *need* to feel good.

When we think of pampering, our minds immediately turn to indulgence at the spa: massage, facial, pedicure. A spa day is the pinnacle of pampering. But you don't have to plan such a lavish treat to be pampered (although, we won't stop you if you do).

The point is to do something to make yourself feel special. A small fortune isn't necessary; neither is a lot of time. Think about the little things that make you feel good. A favorite scent? Bring it to your office in the form of a candle or cream for a spa mini moment. Fresh flowers? Pick up a bouquet with your milk and bread. A good read? Don't leave it on your nightstand; carry it with you so that when you're stuck in the carpool line you can escape the stress of the wait with your fictional fantasy. Relaxing sounds? In this age of downloads, the music that moves you is always at your fingertips. This can turn housework into a dance party. Truly, it is the small things—they add up.

Obviously if you can have someone else pamper you, all the better. Find a willing recruit for a foot rub, call for take-out, take a pass on doing the dishes, and sip a glass of wine or a cup of tea on the porch instead. Watch the sun go down.

Vacation

Vacation \vā-'kā-shən\: Escaping the demands of everyday life for a week, weekend, day, or hour. Recharging your enthusiasm for the "mundane" by checking out for a finite amount of time. Retreat.

Remember that first vacation you took with kids along? Remember how, before you left, you actually believed it would be a vacation? Of course, as soon as you arrived at your destination you realized that no matter where you are—even a beach paradise—you are still on duty.

So obviously, we're not talking about the family vacation. Just like pampering yourself, taking a vacation can be on such a small scale as not to seem worth it, but as we already mentioned, the little things add up. Think about lifting weights. Thirty minutes in the gym isn't likely to yield noticeable results, but keep at it and you'll see and feel the difference in a matter of months.

We're certain that a few days away with your spouse or on a girls' trip will help you get your groove back. But let's face it, we don't always have those plane tickets in hand when the need to escape strikes.

The other problem with getting away sans kids is the production required to make sure the kids are in good hands while you're away. After all that preparation, you really do need a vacation. Same applies if you work outside the home.

So get away, without *going* away. A minimalist escape can be an afternoon alone at your favorite coffee shop, movie theater, or park. Make them easy, accessible getaways so you can actually retreat when you need to. Of course, one of our favorite ways to retreat is on a long walk, run, or bike ride. Taking a yoga class is like a pampering, meditative, active mini vacation. It's the multitasking mama's favorite retreat.

> Recently I left my family one night under the guise that I needed to work. I didn't. I went to see a movie alone. Shhhh. Don't tell.
>
> —Kara

Intimacy

Intimacy \ˈin-tə-mə-sē\: Closeness or familiarity between two people. Feeling connected to someone.

When life's pace leaves little time to spend in bed it may be hard to remember how you got those children in the first place. Those midnight hours aren't filled with romance and mystery. Nope, they become a little war zone in which you fight for the freedom of sleep and await the battle cry down the hall—whether it's nursing babies, toddlers with night terrors, or angst-ridden teenagers.

It's not always that your libido has disappeared—just the ambition to make that first move. When it comes to making a workout happen, fit moms understand that getting started is the hardest part. Get through the first few steps and you quickly remember why you set out to sweat in the first place. Tired sex is like that, too. Remember how good it feels when you're done and you're more motivated to start.

But this section isn't just about hitting the sack. True, sex is a wonderfully restorative form of intimacy, but it isn't quite the same as holding hands, dreams shared, and quiet conversation.

Feeling intimate, that "we're on the same team" feeling, with our spouse or partner does wonders for our mental health. Sharing a life together, as complicated and challenging as it can be, provides substantial benefits in the way of happiness and longevity.

This intimacy isn't limited to a spouse or partner. Sisters, friends, cousins, and parents can all provide us with an intimate, nurturing relationship—a connection that sustains us and provides purpose and support to our life. This is our safety net. Even strong women need one.

These relationships are a vital part of who we are—so much so that we've devoted the next secret to the people who influence and support us. We want them on our fit journey as cheerleaders or partners in fitness; otherwise we have to learn to do it on our own. But we can't finish this section about our body without addressing hormones first. They're kind of like the people in our life, too: can't live with 'em, can't live without 'em.

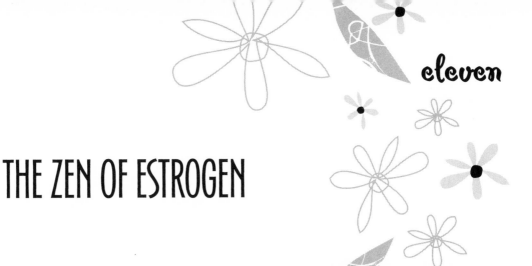

eleven

THE ZEN OF ESTROGEN

We've all experienced their impish wrath. No, we're not talking about your kids. We're talking about hormones. You can't see them. You can't touch them. But you know they're there. Estrogen, in particular, separates the girls from the women and the women from the men. Girls and men produce estrogen, too, but not the copious amount produced by women of reproductive age.

Estrogen's most obvious role in a woman's body is its part in the menstrual cycle (or its disappearing act in the case of menopause). The word *estrogen* comes from the Latin word *estrus*, which means—we're not kidding—"frenzy." Frenzies aside, there's a lot that estrogen does for your body, such as prod your metabolism, help form bones, and work to keep cholesterol ratios in a healthy balance (which is why all three of these areas suffer after menopause). Of course, estrogen is also responsible for making us the shorter sex, making us more prone to constipation, and putting us at risk for certain cancers.

But estrogen doesn't work alone; many other hormones ebb and flow in our bodies, sometimes surging and retreating, sometimes hitting like a tsunami, sometimes disappearing into a black hole. Wouldn't it make you crazy to orchestrate all that? Oh, right, it does. Well, finding the Zen of estrogen, or any hormone harmony for that matter, is possible (just don't expect a miracle, sister), particularly when it comes to the hallmarks of our life: menstruation, pregnancy, and menopause.

Menstruation: Cycling Through Your Cycle

It's easy to fall into a vicious cycle, letting that monthly visitor dictate whether or not you have the mojo to work out. You can't stop the symptoms Mother Nature dishes up for you each month, but there are things you can do so they don't stop you from swimming or running or golfing or even cycling your way through your cycle.

Cramps

As if you didn't suffer enough during childbirth. Sometimes menstrual cramps can make you feel like you're back in labor. Blame your discomfort on a hormonelike substance called prostaglandin. Produced in excess during menstruation, prostaglandins are chemicals that cause contractions in smooth muscle tissue resulting in those painful uterine cramps.

About half of all menstruating females get menstrual cramps on a regular basis. Yes, they hurt, but they shouldn't keep you from exercising. In fact, exercise is the best remedy for cramps. As you already know, your body releases endorphins when you engage in aerobic exercise—anything that gets your heart rate up for at least thirty minutes. These endorphins are your body's natural pain reliever and can keep those prostaglandins in check. When PMS strikes, fight back. Go exercise. Trust us, you'll suffer more if you lie down and take it.

Here are a few other combat techniques to fight off menstrual cramps:

- *Reach for a bottle of nonsteroidal anti-inflammatories (NSAIDs), such as ibuprofen.* But do it before the pain gets bad, and keep up with the dosage on your worst days. NSAIDs will relieve pain and inhibit the production of prostaglandins in the body. Taking them will simultaneously treat both cause and symptom.
- *Make sure you are getting adequate amounts of calcium and magnesium.* Calcium helps maintain normal muscle tone and prevents cramps and pain; magnesium is a natural muscle relaxer and optimizes your body's calcium absorption. Good food sources for magnesium include beans, whole grains, salmon, shrimp, tofu, vegetables, and nuts. Look for calcium-magnesium supplements.
- *Consider avoiding red meats and full-fat dairy products during your premenstrual period.* Research has found that women who followed a low-fat, vegetarian diet for two menstrual cycles experienced less pain and bloating and decreased premenstrual symptoms than those who ate meat. The fat seems to be the culprit here, so choose low-fat dairy products and lean meats or substitute fish and eggs for meat products. Several studies have also reported less menstrual pain with a higher intake of omega-3 fatty acids, which can help reduce inflammation.

Bloating

You may not be pregnant anymore, but sometimes you look like you are. Bloating doesn't just make your jeans uncomfortable—it can be painful, even debilitating. Plus it's hard to work out when your stomach is stretched and taut like a balloon. Make a few changes to your diet to alleviate bloating so you can work out in comfort.

- *Eat small meals throughout the day.* Big meals are just going to make you feel, well, big. Think small portions that provide lasting energy such as whole grains, fruits, and vegetables.

- *Make dietary changes gradually.* Sometimes a sudden increase in fiber from vegetables, fruits, and beans can cause bloating.

- *Consume foods rich in potassium.* Potassium helps you excrete sodium and excess water, thereby reducing that bloated feeling.

- *Stay hydrated.* The more water you consume the less you retain, and the less water you consume the more you retain.

- *Avoid sugary snacks.* We understand, firsthand, the need to stuff your face with cookies, brownies, ice cream, or other yummy foods during "that time of the month." But too much sugar, like too much salt, will make your PMS worse. In addition, refined sugar has a tendency to cause extreme energy highs followed by periods of low energy. None of us wants an energy crash.

- *Cut back or completely cut out alcohol and soda out of your diet,* particularly if you are prone to bloating. Alcohol and soda have a tendency to cause water retention due to high levels of sodium, making bloating worse.

- *Curb your carbs at night.* A carbohydrate-rich meal late at night will cause you to retain fluid. Save that pasta for lunch.

> **Watch your reaction to sugarless gum. Most contain sorbitol, which can cause seriously painful bloating in large amounts. One piece of gum and I'm OK; chew a whole pack and I can barely button my pants.**
>
> —Laurie

Energy Drain

You're already tired, so when your period hits the exhaustion can become unbearable, especially if you have heavy menstrual cycles, which can cause anemia. If you are prone to anemia make sure your multivitamin includes iron (some don't) and load up on iron-rich foods. Make a spinach salad a staple in your diet and snack on dried apricots, raisins, and prunes. Another sure bet: Wash down a tablespoon of molasses with a chug of orange juice.

Fatigue can also be the product of an under- or overactive thyroid. If fatigue persists, ask your doctor to check your thyroid and test you for anemia.

Mood Swings

Truth be told, temper tantrums aren't just for preschoolers. We've all had them. Most of us never get used to the emotional ups and downs that accompany the menstrual cycle. Neither do our families. Don't skip your workouts when you're feeling moody or depressed due to PMS. You know how a workout can subdue a bad mood and relieve stress, so exercise during your period is even more beneficial. Just getting out the door to begin your workout may take extra motivation, but odds are once you're out there you'll be glad you went.

> The last time I had blood work done for fatigue, my physician ordered a vitamin D check along with hemoglobin and thyroid tests. Turns out I was deficient in vitamin D, despite daily outdoor runs all year long. Low vitamin D levels are associated with fatigue; popping that tiny pill each morning has done wonders.
>
> —Laurie

Pregnancy: Heavy with (Hormones and) Child

Being pregnant does not necessarily mean fitness gets benched for nine months. No way. Staying fit during pregnancy is important. Provided your pregnancy is not high-risk, working out is important to the health of both you and your baby and even provides a few perks that inactive moms-to-be miss out on.

We'd tell you to check with your doctor first, but sadly much of the available information regarding exercise during pregnancy cites outdated guidelines (prior to 1994) from the American College of Obstetrics and Gynecology (ACOG) that advised women to keep their heart rates below 140 beats per minute. ACOG changed their guidelines in 2002, dropping the heart rate restrictions and promoting exercise during pregnancy, recommending that pregnant women exercise for at least thirty minutes a day up to seven days a week, just like their nonpregnant counterparts. If your obstetrician missed that memo, go to your next appointment armed with the ACOG pamphlet called "Exercise During Pregnancy," which you can find at http://www.acog.org/.

If you don't know already, find out if your physician or midwife supports your active lifestyle. There might be good reasons to avoid exercise during pregnancy (more on that below) but if your provider is basing decisions on outdated, overly conservative guidelines you should find someone else to monitor your pregnancy so you can discuss your intentions in an open, nonjudgmental atmosphere.

If you wear a heart-rate monitor when you work out, put it away for a while. In the first trimester your blood volume doubles, and your heart is working hard just to pump all that new blood through your body. Your vascular system needs time to accommodate all the extra blood. That's why walking up a flight of stairs spikes most pregnant women's heart rates well above 140, even if the perceived effort doesn't amount to much. In the last trimester, your body has sorted out its blood-flow issues, but by then you might be 20, 30, 40, yes, possibly even 50 pounds heavier. At that point, walking up that flight of stairs is laborious for other reasons.

So don't worry about a number; just exercise at a moderate level. Of course, this will vary from woman to woman. The "talk test" is a great tool to keep yourself in check. If you can't converse with your workout buddy or sing along to your iPod, slow it down.

Doctors know that exercise is equally important for the pregnant body and mind. True, anything a woman does to make her feel healthy and strong will be helpful both during and after pregnancy. The psychological effects of moderate exercise can instill confidence and prevent depression both preterm and postpartum.

However, there are a few guidelines you should consider while exercising pregnant. Possible contraindications may keep you sidelined, such as severe anemia, high blood pressure, previous preterm labor, or if your baby isn't growing as it should. Be sure to consult your midwife or physician before embarking on a prenatal exercise routine.

If you're cleared for activity, just avoid getting your core body temperature too high—unborn children can't cool themselves through sweating. All this takes is a little common sense: Don't exercise outside in the heat of the day. Hot yoga is not a good option for the blooming belly. Modify your workouts as necessary. Contact sports and activities with a risk of falling may have to wait (and absolutely no scuba diving). Proper hydration is important; it speeds the ability for both mother and baby to stay cool. Dehydration can bring on preterm labor and exacerbate contractions. So drink six ounces of water every fifteen to twenty minutes of exercise and avoid getting to the point of feeling thirsty. (Yes, this may mean you're running to the bathroom in equal increments, but that's a good workout too!)

Of course, you should stop exercising and contact your health care provider immediately if you experience pain, bleeding, faintness, irregular heartbeat, pelvic pain, or difficulty walking while pregnant. Other warning signs that warrant a call to your provider include chest pain, headache, muscle weakness, calf pain or swelling, uterine contractions, decreased fetal movement, or fluid leaking from your vagina.

If it turns out you can't exercise for nine months, so what. It's just nine months. Remember, in the grand scheme of things that's a blip on the motherhood radar. After all, the essence of this book is finding a way to exercise for the next eighteen years or more.

If you can exercise, however, you should. Studies have shown that women who exercise during pregnancy have shorter labors as well as a decreased need for induction and painkillers during labor and delivery, even fewer cesarean deliveries. Interestingly, women who stop exercising midpregnancy experience similar outcomes as women who don't exercise at all. So when you reach thirty-six weeks and wonder what the point of that workout is, now you have the motivation.

And what of those hormones? Among the many hormone surges we experience during pregnancy, estrogen soars one thousand times higher than prepregnancy levels, which may explain why we're reduced to tears during that baby powder commercial. Pregnancy can make PMS feel like a bad hair day. As we mentioned earlier, exercise helps us tolerate a number of those ugly side effects, including those endured during pregnancy.

If you need another reason for you to get your growing belly on the move, consider this: Exercise may help prevent and treat gestational diabetes, too. And how does this relate to hormones? Well, hormones in the placenta help your baby grow, but they also block insulin in your body, too. It's called insulin resistance and it means Mom is left with high levels of glucose in her body—also called hyperglycemia. Exercise helps us use that glucose without extra insulin, which is a pretty compelling reason to work out.

> My fitness was a huge plus during labor and delivery; not just physically. I used the same mental focus to work through each contraction as to complete the final miles of a marathon. My doctor had me reach down to feel baby's head—that was all the motivation I needed. One more push and she was out.
>
> —Laurie

As we've continued to state throughout this book, all this exercise isn't just for you. Even when you're pregnant, your exercising body is doing your child good. Specifically, by getting your heart rate up, you help your baby better tolerate episodes of lower oxygen, such as during the birth process. Exercise readies the baby for the stress of birth. Another perk of exercise is found in the placenta. Exercising moms have placentas that grow faster and with more blood vessels, which translates into a bigger "dinner plate" for baby.

But the mental benefits are there, too. Women who know their physical and mental limits and who have worked out during pregnancy are also more likely to go into labor feeling confident and ready to face its demands. Several months of training go into the preparation of running a marathon, which takes most people three to five hours to complete. Considering labor usually lasts much longer than that, it makes sense that women should "train" for labor as an intense physical and mental event.

MOM 2 MOM

With both pregnancy and breast-feeding I was at someone else's beck and call. I exercise to know my own body again after it has been through these huge changes, to embrace this new me.

—Janna, mom of four
Calgary, Alberta

Postpartum: The Fourth Trimester

Postpartum exercise helps restore a new mother's sense of identity, particularly if she was athletic before pregnancy. It helps women shed the extra weight gained during pregnancy, maintain cardiovascular fitness, and improve mental stability. Physically fit moms generally recover more quickly from childbirth both mentally and physically than unfit moms.

Of course, wait until your body is ready before getting back at it. ACOG notes that the physiologic effects of pregnancy can persist for up to six weeks postpartum, longer if you had a complicated pregnancy or delivery, and advises a gradual return to fitness. Be honest with yourself, and remember, we are all different.

By the time I had my third baby I was wise to the fact I didn't need to resume my prepregnancy exercise routine as fast as possible. Sure I took walks to keep my mood lifted, but any more than that I found I would get knocked down by mastitis. Plus, I admit, I preferred to gaze lovingly into my newborn's eyes. By six months, though, I was mentally and physically ready to ramp up the intensity and frequency of my workouts.

—Kara

Most important, whatever you decide to do, make sure that your exercise is stress reducing, not stress inducing. For more about the types of exercise you can do after delivery, check out chapter 16.

Moms suffering from the "baby blues" and even postpartum depression benefit from exercise, but again, only if the benefits outweigh the stress of fitting those workouts in. It's the rapid drop of estrogen and progesterone after childbirth that can bring Mom's spirits down. The affect hormones have on our mood postpartum is similar to what we experience during our period, only one hundred times worse.

Remember how we said exercise helps fight those mood fluctuations during your period? Well, as hard as it may be to get moving, if your mood is suffering, consider exercise your first line of defense for depression. Just remember to talk to your doctor about how to best manage postpartum blues or depression; exercise may be only part of a successful treatment plan.

If you're breast-feeding, you've got to plan your exercise around feeding and/or pumping. Avoid the discomfort of engorged breasts by working out after you feed or pump. While reports have circulated that some infants do not like milk offered after exercise, presumably because of lactic acid in their mother's milk, a 2002 study in *Pediatrics* found that "moderate or even high-intensity exercise during lactation doesn't impede infant acceptance of breast milk."

> **Plunked down on the curb at the finish line of a marathon, neither of my girls had any problems with postworkout nursing. As infants, both girls were used to my marathon training and were eager to nurse right there at the finish.**
>
> —Laurie

In fact, another study, this one from the American College of Sports Medicine, found that women who performed a combination of aerobic exercise and strength training (especially strength training) three times a week were better able to hold on to their bone density. This is good news because, while nursing, a mom doesn't just let down her milk, she also gives away up to 200 milligrams of calcium from her own bones. So take extra calcium and pump iron.

As you increase your activity level, be vigilant about increasing your hydration. You know how much fluid you need to take in to keep up with the demands of breast-feeding.

If you're losing fluid through your sweat, take that into account, too. Our best advice is to drink until your urine runs clear.

Remember, too, that the increased levels of the hormone relaxin that coursed through your body during pregnancy take up to a year after birth before completely going back to prepregnancy levels. Relaxin loosens tendons and ligaments so that your bones can shift to allow your little darling to pass through the birth canal, but it can also make you more prone to pull a muscle or overextend a joint. Be mindful of your limits.

As with all mothering advice, experiment with what works best for you and your baby and take care getting back into regular workout routines. Don't be frustrated by seemingly decreased endurance levels. In the grand scheme of things, it all comes back very quickly.

Menopause: Here in a Hot Flash

Menopause is the only time you can get hot and sweaty with no effort. You'd rather "earn" your sweat, though, wouldn't you? No one enjoys the uncomfortable symptoms associated with menopause, which along with those hot flashes include lethargy, night sweats, insomnia, bladder changes, weight gain, headaches, joint pain, heart palpitations, irritability, depression, and anxiety. Wow, all that to look forward to, huh? This crescendo of symptoms occurs when our ovaries cease to make estrogen, progesterone, and testosterone. This definitely isn't the time to cease your fitness regimen. Regular exercise can reduce and help us manage many of those symptoms.

As women age, decreased hormone levels cause their metabolisms to slow down, resulting in weight gain. Much of that fat gets deposited around the midsection, making women more at risk for heart disease. Women who manage their weight with exercise, including weight-bearing exercise, change

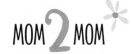

I row, I bike, I run, I swim, I move—somehow, some way. When you are older (and menopausal), you can feel you are fading. Exercise makes me strong and happy. I build an active life and then it compels me to be vibrant in it.

—Annie, mom of three
Northfield Center, Ohio

When I got passed by a fifty-eight-year-old woman at my first triathlon I felt inspired to be that woman twenty years from now!

—Kate, mom of two,
plus two stepchildren
Indianola, Iowa

their muscle-to-fat ratio, increasing their metabolic rate and burning calories in the process. Even at rest. How's that for efficiency?

In our thirties, we women lose about 1 percent of our bone mass each year. During menopause, that rate increases up to 3 percent per year. By exercising regularly, however, we can actually increase bone density and decrease the risk of osteoporosis.

With the infusion of endorphins, regular exercise can also hold back headaches and joint pain, elevate mood, boost energy, and improve sleep.

Can hormone therapy do all that? For some women, exercise truly is the best medicine. Even the North American Menopause Society states, "Exercise may cause the same magnitude of change as that induced by estrogen therapy." We like that endorsement, of course. So, shoot for daily exercise, but try to get it in before the evening hours. Exercising too close to bedtime is yet another trigger for night sweats.

Here are a few things you can do to alleviate those pesky hot flashes, so you're not too hot to work up an exercise-induced sweat:

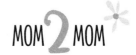

- *Identify and avoid your triggers.* Determine what it is that causes your hot flashes and take note to avoid or alleviate those situations in the future. Is it stress, anxiety, or certain foods? Common triggers to look for include alcohol, caffeine, smoke, spicy or hot foods, warm weather, and hot rooms or showers.

> I hope that in old age I will be able to keep up with not only my kids but also my grandkids. I want to be the fun grandma!
>
> —Becky, mom of one
> Savage, Minnesota

- *Dress appropriately.* Just as you should avoid wearing cotton during workouts, think of your hot flashes as spontaneous workouts (the glass is half full, right?). Choose clothing made of wicking materials such as CoolMax and Dri-FIT. Just another good reason to put on those cute workout clothes, whether or not you intend to exercise. Some companies even make menopause pajamas made of moisture-wicking fabrics.
- *Reduce fat.* That applies to your plate as well as your body. A low-fat diet as well as a low-fat body alleviates hot flashes for some women. Keep enough fat on your body to stay healthy; being underweight can have a negative impact in this department, too.
- *Get your vitamin E.* Some research suggests that taking up to 800 IU on a daily basis will decrease how often and how severe those hot flashes and night sweats are during menopause and perimenopause. There's a bonus here, too—vitamin E also strengthens

the immune system and may protect the heart in those who don't already have cardiovascular disease. Check with your doctor to see if such a high dosage is right for you.

■ *Experience the joy of soy.* Some research suggests that soy may help alleviate hot flashes and other symptoms of menopause. Try soy foods, instead of supplements. Good sources include soy milk, tofu, tempeh, miso, and whole soybeans.

Getting and staying in shape can help you get and stay in charge of your hormones. Show those little dictators who is boss. And maintain command when the external forces of life start to pull at you, too. The stronger you are (physically, mentally, hormonally), the more likely you are to create a supportive environment to help you and your family grow in fitness. Now let's take a look at what you can do to tackle the barrage of *external* forces that come your way.

Secret Number Four

PEOPLE CAN
SABOTAGE YOUR
FITNESS FASTER THAN
A COOKIE BINGE

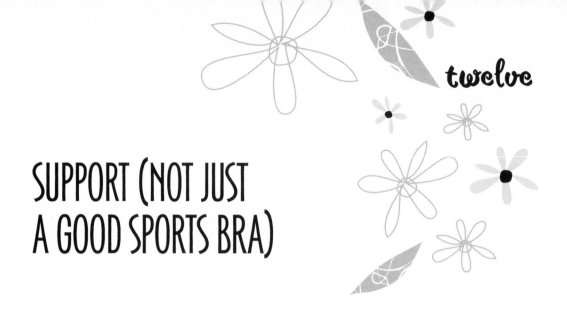

twelve

SUPPORT (NOT JUST A GOOD SPORTS BRA)

Have you ever set the alarm for an early morning workout, but before getting out of bed you heard a voice: "Don't do it. Stay in bed. It's warm and cozy. You need the sleep." Sometimes the voice you hear is your own. Sometimes, though, the voice is real and is coming from a warm body snuggled up next to you.

Even the most dedicated women can struggle to get in their workouts. With children to raise, careers to build, homes to manage, and all the other little things that life throws our way, fitness can sometimes feel like a square peg in a world of round holes. But the kicker is sometimes it's the people closest to us that make things more difficult: a partner, children, a friend, coworker, siblings, or even a parent, who might subtly or not so subtly disapprove.

Make no mistake, you don't need anyone's approval to get and stay fit. However, having a support network can certainly make things easier and even enjoyable.

How to Gain Support from Your Cheering Squad

Let's assume your support system is in equilibrium; you're not feeling disapproval, per se, but you're not getting much encouragement to work out, either. Gaining support doesn't start on the defensive. It doesn't start with an argument about "higher living," or even opening the lines of communication by politely asking for more support. It's important not to seek out change from your future cheering squad, because this isn't about changing them, it's about changing you. This is about *your* actions. Here are some ways to attract support, or at least how *not* to repel it.

Respect Time

Living a fit lifestyle requires that you take time to pursue fitness. As we've already discussed in previous chapters it's not easy finding this time in our day. Often, to acquire said time, we have to "borrow" it from somewhere—or someone—else.

Say you like to run on your lunch hour. That doesn't mean you have an hour to run. You have to factor time to get in and out of your running clothes and time to eat (this is part of the fit equation, too). If you're a quick-change artist you might be able to squeeze in forty-five minutes, at best, so that you don't take advantage of your employer (or worse, piss off the other employees who stick to their allotted hour for lunch).

The same applies to your family. If your plan is to work out on Saturday morning, make certain that you don't leave your partner or kids in a lurch. Assume that your partner has things to do, too, and stick to the plans you've made. Make it to that soccer game if you promised your daughter you'd be there. In order to accomplish everything you've promised (to yourself and to your family), you might have to get up earlier than you'd like to on a Saturday morning. You might have to decline the invitation to go out for pancakes with your pals.

Once we overcome feeling guilty about being away from our families or friends, once we realize we really do deserve the time to ourselves, it's easy to cross the line and feel entitled to more. Getting in a little "me time" can be intoxicating; often we want to overindulge. It's like money—there's never enough. Resist that dangerous mindset. Enjoy your "me time," but don't overdo it.

MOM 2 MOM

I do a boot camp workout over my lunch hour at work. I don't have time to do a full shower and get ready, so after a quick rinse and blow-dry through sweaty hair I'm back at my desk. Prior to being a mom I never would have done that but it's the only way I can fit my workout in now.

—Alicia, mom of two
Chaska, Minnesota

Avoid Overtalking

Once we've made fitness a "habit," there is a certain sense of pride and excitement about accomplishing new and perhaps more lofty goals. We know how exciting it can be to go farther, faster, higher, or longer than we ever have before. It feels good to win a game, hit a home run, lift a heavier weight, or score a goal. These milestones impact your confidence in big ways. And it feels wonderful to share your accomplishments and your passion for fitness with those around you. Just don't be smug about it. Sometimes exercise enthusiasts turn people off with their fervor. We want our passion to be contagious, not lethal to our friendships.

By all means share "your best workout ever," how you've lost more weight, or your secret to boundless energy (for sure, we want to know about that one). When you do, though, be mindful of just exactly how much the other person wants to hear, take time to let them respond, and—this is important—take time to listen.

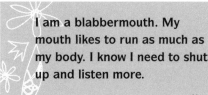

I am a blabbermouth. My mouth likes to run as much as my body. I know I need to shut up and listen more.

—Kara

Show Your Gratitude

The reality is, as mothers, we're always on borrowed time. Someone always wants us somewhere else. The trick is not to resent it, but to be grateful—truly grateful—for the time we get just to ourselves. We're not saying you should be grateful in a generic sense, either, but *express your gratitude directly* to those who make it possible. Let your boss know how much you love to run during your lunch hour (perhaps add how running increases your afternoon productivity). Let your kids know how happy you feel after a workout. Tell your partner how much you appreciate the time you get on the weekends for fitness. You get the point. You teach your children good manners; make sure you lead by example. Say thank you.

Returning the Favors

The only thing better than saying thank you is *showing* your gratitude. The most direct way of doing this is by giving time back to those people who help support your fit lifestyle. That means willingly, happily, and encouragingly saying, "Have fun" when your partner wants to get in his workout (or walk the aisles of Home Depot, or play chess, or whatever it is he does). With your children, this might mean taking them on a bike ride of their own when you're through with yours, or letting them hit a bucket of balls with you at the driving range. At work you might stay a little later in the day if you take extra time at lunch to exercise. It's not so much about making sacrifices for others as it is making "deposits" into the Bank of Nice. Karma, people. It's about karma.

Why People Try to Sabotage Your Fitness

Sadly, even when you're exuding respect and gratitude for the people around you, it doesn't always work in your favor. Sometimes people live in a house of mirrors, so they only see themselves. It's unfortunate, especially when such people are important to you. They might make it difficult for you to get your workouts in or induce guilty feelings for taking the time to exercise. Maybe they say things like, "Why do you need to exercise?" or "What a waste of time!" so that you question your priorities. Maybe it's a more passive-aggressive reaction. Sometimes it helps to understand why people might react to your fitness in such ways.

Jealousy

There you are sweating off the pounds, buffing up your arms, perhaps entering races. The strength you've gained physically exudes in your every move, down to the twinkle in your eye and the smile on your face. You feel good. You don't have to tell anyone; they can see it. Perhaps your sister sees it and can't be happy for you because she doesn't have (but wants) both your look and feel.

It can be difficult to own up to jealousy. More often the ugly green monster lashes out as anger, snide remarks, or hurtful actions. Nobody wants to admit they're not taking care of themselves the way they'd like, can see (in you) how it's being done successfully, but can't get over their bitterness to say: "Hey, I like the way you're living. Can you help me have what you have?"

The envy may not be over your strong arms, your weight loss, or your speed. Perhaps it's over the new relationships you've discovered with like-minded people. Maybe your husband is feeling a little out of sorts because there are new people in your life that you're spending time with (while you run, jump, ride, climb, swim, and so forth).

Fear

The people close to you might genuinely feel they are losing you to a new love. If fitness is relatively new and becomes a "passion," this aura of new love isn't entirely off base. In addition, if your body has been through a metamorphosis because of exercise, your spouse may fear that the "you" inside has changed, too, which it probably has because you're stronger, more powerful, more confident, and more motivated than ever before. Anyone who doesn't feel that way about his or her own self might be intimidated. They might fear losing you altogether.

Selfishness

Sometimes it happens that the people in your life may not want what you have, but they don't want you to have it, either. This most often manifests in battles over your time. It may seem to your partner that you're choosing a workout over spending time with him, even if he's spending that time, say, lying on the couch watching a hockey game. You may get this from your kids, who have no concept of boundaries on your time. This you expect, of course. It's harder to deal with when it's an adult. It's hard to be patient. It's hard to see what's happening with an empathetic lens.

Various forms of sabotage may go on with other aspects of your healthy lifestyle, such as in the nutritional arena. If you're eating healthier, you may find your coworkers enticing you with doughnuts in the break room or fat-laden lunches. "You're too skinny!" you might hear them say. What they're really saying is: "I'm too fat, please join me!" Family dinners may take on a similar tone with protests about healthier meals. Don't take "yuck" personally. Stand firm; this is one battle you want to win.

MOM 2 MOM

My husband has tried about everything to make me want to give up running: arguments, not speaking to me, purposely planning stuff when he knows I've made arrangements already, jokes that I never win, the cost of it. So I feel I have to hide it from him. Like an affair. I get up early or I wait until he leaves. I sometimes lie about it and I feel bad but I try to keep the peace. I also feel bad that I'm not setting a very good example to my kids. I don't want them to think it's normal to do that in a relationship. I tell them that they need to find someone who loves and supports them wholly.

—Connie, mom of four
Carroll, Iowa

Tactics for Turning the Tables

Keep your radar up and notice when you're feeling defensive about your fit lifestyle. Oftentimes the people who try to sabotage our fitness leave us feeling like we need to justify our workouts to them, and to ourselves. They may be passive-aggressive and initiate an argument on some unrelated front—the kind of argument that leaves you wondering, "What is this really about?" They may poke playful jabs at you, but their jokes leave you feeling wounded even after the conversation moves on. Or, you might be confronted more directly and end up in an argument.

It's important to avoid engaging in arguments with people who express themselves this way. If the relationships are meaningful to you, then saying "You're just jealous!" or "You're being selfish!" probably isn't the best response, even though it may be the truth. Instead, look at the situation from their perspective and figure out the real source of their discontent. It never hurts to take a long look within, too. Consider whatever accusations you've been dealt. Is there any truth to what's been said?

It's important to let people know that pursuing a fit life is a priority to you. Take the time to discuss exactly why. Now is also a good time to explain how meaningful their relationship is to you, too, and that you'd like their support, maybe even their company, during your next workout.

However, here's a big disclaimer: If your passion for fitness has crossed from priority to obsession, then your cheering squad may be raising red flags. If you can't go a day without working out, if you routinely choose workouts over family obligations, or your compulsion to exercise interferes with responsibilities at home or work, then it may not be lack of support you feel, but intervention from your cheering squad.

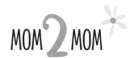

MOM 2 MOM

Without telling my husband, I woke up extra early and set out to run 26.2 miles. By myself. On a hot day. With just a single water bottle. After I finished, I came home to find him very upset about my long absence. I couldn't be bothered with that, though, as I had to make it to my kickboxing class. My husband said there was no way I was going and took the car keys. I was so intent on my workout that I dug out the spare key and took all the kids to the gym anyhow. I still had not had anything to eat or drink. I barely finished the class before I fainted. My husband was waiting for me when we got home and that was the beginning of the intervention. It wasn't long after that I found myself in eating disorder therapy for compulsive overexercise.

—Charlotte, mom of four
Lakeville, Minnesota

What to Do When You Don't Get Support

While we've focused on people in our inner circle, sometimes people we don't know can do or say things that make us feel awful (or conversely, really great, with a simple "Way to go!"). When it comes to avoiding negative comments by strangers, we hope you can shake your head and shrug it off.

As for relationship trials and tribulations with family and friends, we hope you're a brilliant diplomat. Sometimes as gracious as we try to be, nothing works. As you already know, you can't change people; you can only change the way you react to them (and then hope they come around). But if they don't soften up, open up, or join you, then you have a choice to make. When you run into resistance from the people closest to you, and realize that the resistance is there to stay, there are two paths you can follow.

Avoid Emotional Vampires

We tell our children to avoid playing with kids who do or say things that make them feel bad. It's time to heed that advice and realize that some relationships require more energy to maintain than you're willing to give. This doesn't mean you are a bad person; it means you've properly applied your values to your relationships. In general, it's never a good idea to surround yourself with negative people. These emotional vampires can suck the joy right out of your life. If you've worked to attract their support and there's no good vibe, you're better off limiting contact so you don't get pulled down into the mire. Sometimes it's not necessarily the people you have to avoid, just certain topics. Know what they are and avoid them.

MOM 2 MOM

I once took my kids out to a playground and ran laps around the structure so I could keep an eye on them. While I was running my laps I had another mother (sitting on her blanket texting) approach me with accusations of neglect (everything from her having to supervise my children to being selfish for exercising instead of watching my kids). This made me doubt myself as a good mother. I have since come to terms with this incident and concluded that I am a fantastic mother to my two girls but I am realistic about needing to fit time in for me during my hectic day. Most important, no one should question or judge what another woman needs or does in her life.

—Lori, mom of two
Spruce Grove, Alberta

Let It Go

Another way to handle the negativity is to thicken your skin, tune it out, and let it go. When someone encourages you to skip a workout or questions your commitment to fitness, tune it out with your own mantra. Let your eyes glaze over. Smile and nod and in your head, repeat something like: "I am strong. I am a lioness. I could eat you right now!" Seriously, though, if you expect negative comments on a regular basis from certain people, have a line ready and waiting in the wings, so you're not left feeling punched in the gut every time you see them. Something like: "I'm sorry you feel that way. My workouts are a priority for me because I want to lead a healthy life for me and for my family." Accepting, rather than changing, these people is the key to keeping your relationship healthy. Don't get sucked in. Breathe. And when you exhale, let it go.

Changing your body on the outside is hard work. But to do it effectively requires you take a look at the things on the inside, too. While you are dropping pounds and getting cut, you must also slice through some of your mental hang-ups to set boundaries for yourself, garner support from those around you, nurture your healthy friendships, and see other friendships for what they really are.

Now it's time to look a bit closer at our relationships with our significant others. Read on to discover just how fitness helps bring couples closer together and how to jump the hurdles that drive couples apart.

> My parents and siblings don't quite understand why my husband and I run like we do. After taking a few jabs, we've learned to avoid talking about it too much. It's now on our hush-hush list, along with religion and politics.
>
> —Laurie

thirteen

THE SWEAT ON SIGNIFICANT OTHERS

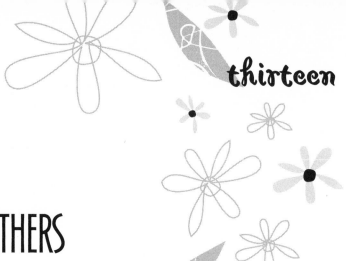

Everyone brings baggage into a relationship. If you're lucky it might be a little, tiny change purse. Others seem to drag along the entire line of Samsonite. If fitness is part of your life, then you at least carry your gym bag.

We're not suggesting your love for fitness is some sort of baggage; but, like forgetting to put the cap on the toothpaste, it can muddy marital bliss if you're not careful. Your athletic aspirations have a certain magnetism about them, and how you pursue them determines which end of the magnets you're putting together and whether they will attract or repel your mate.

Because it's not always easy to find time for quality moments with your honey, it becomes especially difficult to slip out of a warm bed at 5 a.m. to run in the dead of winter. And if your husband likes early morning workouts, too, those days of snuggling up like twisted pretzels under the covers can become a faint memory. The other side of the day isn't necessarily easier. Leaving for the gym the minute he walks in the door makes that "Honey, I'm home!" kiss feel like a baton in life's relay.

Regardless of your spouse's athletic ambitions, at the end of the day, he could probably use a little "me"

MOM 2 MOM

There have been times I cannot do my usual early morning run so I've literally run out of the house the second my husband gets home from work in the evening. He's told me numerous times that if he didn't know better, he'd think I was running away from home because I'm out of there so fast.

—Theresa, mom of two
Long Island, New York

time, too. How you balance that—lovingly, willingly, happily—with your need to squeeze in a quick run before dinner is the secret to relationship success. Having this spirit of cooperation is the force that brings those magnets together.

Couples Who Do It Together and Those Who Don't (Work Out, That Is)

As they say, men and women are from different planets. If your partner lives a fit life, too, then at least you're orbiting in the same solar system. You understand each other's need for sweat, personal challenge, and perhaps competition. Still, that doesn't negate the challenges of nurturing your relationship.

And remember that if your partner doesn't share your enthusiasm for fitness, it isn't grounds for divorce. A mutual devotion for the sweaty life might seem incumbent on your success as a fit mom—at least he "gets it"—but that isn't necessarily so. He doesn't have to be fit to love you.

There's a lot of great relationship advice out there, like "make it work." (Nothing like hearing this whispered into your ear by your new mother-in-law at your wedding.) But we're nowhere near qualified to give you relationship advice. We'll leave that to Dr. Phil. But we can tell you how to garner the support of a sedentary spouse, and we can provide tips for keeping "sweat equity" within the relationship if you have a fit spouse.

When She Alone Wears the Running Shorts

As a Hot (Sweaty) Mama, your goal isn't to make him see the error of his nonathletic ways or force him to love what you do. As long as you can be the fit mom you want to be, it simply doesn't matter if he's sweating alongside you.

You don't need to manage him, change him, or coerce him. Now, see? Suddenly you have more energy for your workouts, which otherwise would have been inappropriately used to berate your partner (or stew in an equally damaging passive-aggressive manner). Being fit isn't about *him*. It is about *you*. Are you feeling the built-up layers of frustration peel away from you? We hope the switch in this thought process becomes a huge sanity-saving (perhaps even relationship-saving) revelation. Truly your relationship doesn't need to hinge on a shared passion for fitness. Besides, who cares how he feels about your exercise habits so long as you get your workout in?

Now, getting that workout in will be infinitely easier if you make it easy for him to support you. Think about those magnets again: You want to attract, not repel. If you are lucky enough that your partner acquired the gene to be naturally empathetic and supportive, he is likely already involved to whatever extent you need: whether it be asking you about your training or waiting for you at the finish line with flowers. Most partners, however, may not be so intuitive. Again, we're not suggesting you nudge him in any way. You can only be responsible for you and what you bring to the relationship. We do think the following five rules for the Hot (Sweaty) Mama are nothing more than a considerate approach to loving the one you're with. But, in doing so, we hope it kindles that spirit of cooperation, so that getting out the door for your workout of choice is made easier because *he* wants you to go.

Vow Number One: Do Unto Others

If you want time for fitness, make sure you give him time to pursue his favorite activities, too. You might not be interested in playing poker or fantasy football with the neighborhood guys, but you can still be interested in his involvement. Ask questions, listen, and don't roll your eyes over his excitement. Who knows, you may actually learn to enjoy an afternoon lecture on the subtle nuances of tire changes in the pits of the Daytona 500, or why the pitcher threw a hanging curveball on a 0–2 count to a classic fastball hitter. Basically, we're suggesting you take an interest in his life with the same enthusiasm with which you'd like him to treat your passion for fitness.

MOM 2 MOM

I know I've been an influence on my husband—he's now run four marathons and finished one triathlon. But it's not his thing the way it's my thing. That's fine; I'd rather him do what makes him most happy. That happens to be golf and poker—worlds away from running and triathlons. What allows our "separate lives" to coexist is mutual support and respect for each other's interests. We want each other to have fun (we believe this is paramount in a marriage and in life). Our different interests have made our life together more interesting. Craig definitely set the standard for supporting my interests, so I return the favor, and—this is important—try not to take advantage of it. I'm careful to maintain balance and keep family first.

—Janice, mom of two
Coppell, Texas

Vow Number Two: Sweat Responsibly

Don't take advantage of your training time. If you plan an early morning bike ride and your pals propose hitting the diner for breakfast after, take a pass. Do what you need to do to stay fit but be conservative when it comes to socializing. There will be times you can (and should) plan for a social hour after an event, but stick to the planned schedule. If you said you'd be home by 10 a.m. after your ride, be there.

Vow Number Three: Extend an Invitation

Your partner can be a part of your workout without actually working out himself. Ask him to assist by bringing you food and/or water. Introduce him to your training partners. Take him to a race. Ask him to volunteer. Let him know how important his support is to you. Make sure he knows he plays a big role.

Vow Number Four: Put Him in Charge

What man doesn't want to be in control? Give your partner a task and let him be king of his domain. If you're not a gear head yourself, consider asking your husband to be in charge of bike or other equipment maintenance. Let him figure out how to work that new heart-rate monitor you just bought, or map some new running routes for you on the Internet.

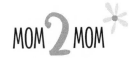

MOM 2 MOM

My husband is my official chip-timer-putter-on guy! I have never put on my own chip for a race.

—Erica, mom of three
Waldorf, Maryland

Vow Number Five: Keep Your End of the Deal

Every couple must divide and conquer household chores. Agree upon a good balance of work. There will be times when you are dead tired, but for the sake of marital bliss, don't shirk your duties. Whether you are treasurer of your family finances or project manager of the laundry mill, don't let these job descriptions get buried under your running clothes. Keep the momentum to keep the peace.

Yes, we're convinced taking on the crusade to transform your spouse into a training partner is not the point. However, your lifestyle might be a beacon toward a healthier way of life. He may not ever turn into a competitive athlete, but you may subtly inspire him to exercise for basic health benefits. Just give him the opportunity to love what you do—even if at a distance.

When You Both Say "I Do" to Fitness

A mutual affection for fitness may be the perfect backdrop for true love, but it's no guarantee for bliss. Mars is still Mars and Venus is still Venus. Sharing the same active lifestyle can present its own set of challenges. Again, a spirit of cooperation must be at play in order to serve each other's athletic needs among the many duties required of a marriage and family. Even though you both value fitness, being self-centered about your own agenda can suck your love life into a black hole.

Vow Number One:
Know Each Other's Training Schedule

If you're headed out the door for a run and realize he left ten minutes ago and no one is around to watch the kids, keep your cool and hold off on retaliation. Yes, he didn't tell you he was leaving for a run, but neither did you. It smacks of a communication problem that likely runs deeper than your fitness plans. Once kids come along you can't always wing it. If you were never one to plan your workout schedule a week or more in advance, now is the time to change. You have to be more meticulous with your planning. If he knows your schedule in advance and inadvertently sneaks out the door before you, then you're free to let him have it!

> When our twins arrived my husband and I both felt entitled to get in our workouts. Finally we concluded neither of us was going to give up our passion so we needed to compromise. What ultimately worked for us was dividing the week, so that we each had designated mornings to work out. On weekends we take turns or use the gym's child care. For the most part this works great, but every now and again we experience a setback. When it comes to communicating we still have training to do.
>
> —Kara

Vow Number Two: Support Each Other

This starts by sharing your goals. Understanding and empathy help us to be better spouses. Know when difficult workouts are on the calendar. You can support his efforts by making his favorite carbo-loading meal the night before or greeting him at the finish line (even if that's your front door) with enthusiasm. Coordinate your race schedule so that some are shared and others are solo adventures. Exchange war stories when you both compete; take advantage of the family support when you go it alone.

Vow Number Three:
Accommodate and Sacrifice

Help each other find time to work out. No, you can't meet your running buddies five nights a week. This means that sometimes you spend part of your weekend getting in your workout while your spouse runs errands with the kids, and then you switch it up. It may also mean that one of you has to get up at hours you didn't know existed to get your workout in.

Vow Number Four: Go on Fitness Dates

Even if you don't move at the same pace you can both head to the same place for a workout and refuel together afterward. Consider team play or group activities if your ability levels are not well matched.

Vow Number Five: Become a Fit Family

Taking the time to work out as a couple is great—now extend the invitation to your children. Let them run alongside the jogger or swim a few laps with you at the pool. Watch them mimic your behavior and love every minute of it. Dedicate some larger chunks of time, too, where everyone is active together. Take a soccer ball to the park or go for a family bike ride. Try something new like orienteering or rock climbing. Just get out there and move. See chapters 15 and 16 for ideas on getting fit as a family.

MOM 2 MOM

We take turns working out: mornings for me, evenings for him. The real struggle is spouse time together.

—Scottie, mom of two
Greenville, North Carolina

Athleticism has always been a big part of my relationship with my husband. After our first daughter was born, we planned long runs around naptime when the baby would be sleeping in the stroller. We ran early in the morning or at lunchtime. We took turns biking to work. When all else failed we enjoyed some evening family time in the form of a run or ride, pushing or pulling our daughters along.

—Laurie

Here's to the Ones We Love

Whether or not they exercise themselves, some partners are super supportive. Others, well, not so much. What camp are you in? Here's what it feels like for moms with significant others on either side of the fence, with those straddling the top and those trying to climb it.

The Kind Who Makes You Say "Ahhhhhh"

- He's the one pushing me out the door to run sometimes. He volunteers to take the kids places so that I can run, or he takes me out trail running because he knows I won't do it alone.

- My husband asks me every day if I had time for a walk, and if I say no, he makes time for me!

- He watches the kids while I work out, has bought me fitness equipment as gifts, gently nudges me out the door when I am not feeling motivated, and commends me for the workouts I've done and improvements I've made in my fitness level. (In return, he gets golf time.)

- He takes care of my son while I go to hockey practices/games and helps find money in the budget for me to be able to buy any fitness equipment I may want or need.

- I love to run to a local park on the weekends, and he and the boys come pick me up and bring me Gatorade, snacks, and so on.

- My husband will cook dinner so that I can work out.

- He encourages me to work out regularly and when I am stressing about exercising versus doing other family stuff, he usually tells me to exercise first! (I think he knows it's in his best interest, too!)

- On "my mornings" to go for a run, he gets up with the baby during the night so I have some rest.

- He allays my guilt about leaving the kids for a while to work out by reminding me how crabby I get if I don't!

- I go to yoga every Sunday. He has been known to say: "Well, we can't do that; it's during your yoga!"

- My husband always used to say "I want to be the kind of family that goes for a run on Saturday mornings." He is holding true to his promise: Rain or shine, we make it out on our Saturday morning runs . . . as a family.
- He tells me how proud he is of me.

The Kind Who Makes You Say "Ewwww"
- My husband regularly makes negative comments about what I do for exercise.
- When I ran my first half marathon, he refused to come. It was really important to me that my children watch me cross the finish line, but my husband wouldn't budge on the issue. He said that he wouldn't give up his first weekend hunting for this. Please note that he hunts frequently and has done so for many years. This was my first half marathon, and my children missed it. It is still very painful for me to think about.
- I get the guilt trip when I take the time to run or work out.
- He controls the finances and there's never enough money for me to race or buy gear, but there's strangely enough money for him to eat out or buy new books. He also complains about the time it takes from the family. Never mind I run before the kids are up, and often take them with me to workouts or even to races (the few times I get to race).
- He feels like it takes time away from him and the family, but he does not see that I get up at 5 a.m. to work out while the house is still sleeping!
- The least he does is roll his eyes. It gets worse from there.

The Kind Who Straddles the Fence
- He totally supports my fitness, especially when I take the kids with me.
- As long as it doesn't interfere with his schedule or make his life more difficult, he is supportive.
- We try to trade off days for the early morning chores. But I get guilt if I try and exercise at night!
- He says he'll help out so I can run but it always seems like when he's finally available I'm exhausted. (We're still talking about exercise, right?)
- He is supportive but refuses to come to races anymore; he says it's brutal trying to entertain the kids for hours while he waits for the chance to see me run past for five seconds.
- He definitely supports my efforts in general but is not a morning person (so I have to handle child care issues myself).

- He doesn't roll his eyes too much when I want to get a new Garmin or pair of running shoes.
- There are times that I can tell he is resentful, but on the other hand, if I don't get a run or exercise in, it makes for a very long day!
- He will encourage me to get out and run if I need to, but I want to see him and my son at the finish line at races (with a sign . . . oh, and maybe a supercute handmade onesie).
- Although my spouse does support my efforts to be fit, it sometimes feels as if *his* efforts to be fit take priority. He gets to exercise at work every day without question, and I always have to "fit in" my exercising: either waiting until he gets home from work, or doing it while my kids are sleeping. And it's a lot harder for me to get my exercising time in without something else coming up.
- My workout times are limited to the morning hours, and tennis practice and challenge matches in the evening seem to cause problems.
- My husband doesn't have an inkling why I am doing this, but he has never tried to discourage me. I find my emotional support online.

The Kind Who Sees the Light

- Although it took a couple months for my husband to get used to me taking time for myself for karate class and one time threatening to take it away (as if he could), he has adapted to the change and has been my biggest cheerleader at competitions.
- As a result of my love for working out he joined a gym and has been exercising as well. He always thought working out would "ruin" his golf swing but I think he's realized it has improved his swing!
- My husband was and is very supportive in my new career as a personal trainer. He even joins in on my boot camp classes.
- I wanted to create a workout room in our home. He was all over the plan and helped me move the rooms around and was even looking for weights and a rack for me.
- Now that he is getting fit, too, we take turns watching the kids so we can get in our workouts.
- My love of running sparked my husband's interest, and now he's coaching marathon groups and training for an ultramarathon this fall. He understands the importance of making the time, so he helps me fit my runs in as well.

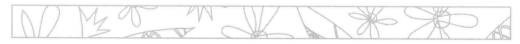

Sex and the Sweaty

Regular exercise leaves you feeling pretty good, doesn't it? Fit, strong, and confident probably fall into your list of personal adjectives. What about horny? If your primal urges rival those of the teenage boy next door, not to worry. Regular exercise can make you hot and, well, bothered. Cardiovascular fitness translates into better circulation—arousal depends on healthy blood flow. Exercise also encourages the production of more sex hormones. Biologically speaking, exercise is an aphrodisiac.

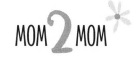

Working out on a regular basis prepares you for a better sex life psychologically, too. The better you know your body, the healthier your self-image, the more likely you are to be pleased (or please yourself). Replace the stress with those feel-good hormones that come with exercise, and you're more likely to be "in the mood" when the lights go down.

Nevertheless, everyone knows that the sacred rite of parenthood can have a diminutive affect on heated moments between the sheets—especially for a fit couple. What are the odds your kids will be banging down the door during a midday quickie attempt? At night, too many readings of *Goodnight Moon* may kill the urge. When the alarm goes off, you make the choice—sleep in, exercise, or nookie.

Hopefully, your hormonal overdrive isn't cause for frustration. Sex *can* be doable, even when you have young children. A good sex life is much like staying fit—it requires motivation and a little ambition. Of course, that applies to all of the things in life we enjoy—whether it's time spent with your spouse, sweating at the gym, engaging in a favorite hobby, or, as we'll see in the next chapter, socializing with friends.

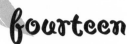

fourteen

THE SWEATY SISTERHOOD

> Athletic female w/kids seeking like-minded training partner to enjoy long walks in park, rural bike rides, inline skating, and other activities. Dependability a must, enthusiasm a plus. Those without a sense of humor need not respond.

Remember your first? Your first really dependable workout partner, that is. In particular, we're talking about a woman with whom you shared a specific fitness goal, interest, or skill. She was someone you could rely on, someone who could rely on you. You had a special bond from which some sort of sisterhood grew.

It's true; sweat opens up more than our pores. It gets us to say things—admit things we might not divulge in normal conversation. Sweat becomes a truth serum that makes us both strong and vulnerable at the same time. For some moms, sharing that sweat with other women means strengthening, deepening, or creating friendships on a level that they haven't experienced since their single days or perhaps never had before.

MOM 2 MOM

Running is a large part of my social life. I have met moms with children older than mine and I gained valuable advice that I can now pass along to moms with younger children. I would have never met some of my best friends otherwise.

—Michele, mom of two
Coppell, Texas

If you're new to fitness, this might sound too good to be true, and maybe it's one more good reason to get yourself off the couch and into those workout clothes. Sweaty sisters don't just get us up and moving—they make workouts fun and add texture to our lives even after we've washed the sweat away. Exercise is more than just a means to a healthy mind and body; it's a path to lasting relationships, social events, and sometimes a group therapy session. Now *that's* multitasking.

Seeking Sweaty Sisters

How on earth do you find these kindred spirits, these new best friends? It might seem a bit like dating. And it is, cause it takes a little effort to find or establish a group of women who have equal amounts of flexibility and dependability, two traits necessary for fit moms who wish to sweat together. Like many of your relationships, these special friendships seem to just appear; the universe simply brings you together. However, if you're desperately seeking a sweaty sister, you might check out a few options.

1. Investigate local clubs or training groups in whatever activities interest you the most. A quick Web search of your city and favorite sport is likely to bring up a group within your vicinity.

2. Enjoy volleyball, soccer, or softball? Join a sports league to find instant teammates.

3. Online networks also help moms team up. At http://www.seemommyrun.com/, you can search your zip code for moms looking for running partners. At http://www.momsinmotion.com/, you can find or start a training group of athletic moms in your area. A Web search will likely turn up other options.

4. Training partners might be right under your nose. Perhaps there are coworkers who would like a lunchtime workout as much as you, or moms who have taxied

> When I was pregnant with my first, I met a couple of really wonderful women on an online forum (blush). We've traveled a number of times with one family and enjoyed sharing workout stories, tips, and training advice. They live about three hundred miles away, but whenever we get together it's like we've been neighbors forever.
>
> —Laurie

their children to lessons and would rather get out for a walk than fiddle through the outdated magazines in the waiting area.

5. When you see the same woman at the gym over and over again, it might not be coincidence. Most new friendships start with "hello."

6. Some personal trainers organize workouts for groups of neighbors in their own backyards. Schedule something like this and see who comes to your sweaty block party.

7. Make a date to exercise with one other mom you know. Chances are, if you're already friends she'll make an ideal sweaty sister—you just need to recruit her to join the fit revolution.

8. Set a goal, start to train, and share your enthusiasm. Like the Pied Piper, you might pick up other willing participants. Some goals to consider are a local fun run or bike tour, but you could create your own "finish line," such as going to twenty group fitness classes in one month.

9. See someone doing that activity you love the most? Talk to her. Ask if you can join her.

10. Get to know the people in your neighborhood or on your training routes. Start up a conversation or ask them to join you for a bit.

> After my mainstay running partner moved to another state I sent an e-mail to neighbors and friends close by asking if they'd be interested in joining me on my morning runs. I wasn't going to run alone and feel sorry for myself. Reminds me of when we moved to a new house when I was eight years old; I went door-to-door looking for friends. I haven't changed much.
>
> —Kara

MOM 2 MOM

I have a girl crush on a mom I see running in town. Actually I am crushing on her whole family: her perfect golden retriever, her perfect running husband, and her cute little boy in their jogging stroller. I really want to stop one day and ask her to be my running partner and to have playdates with us (her son seems to be about the same age as mine).

—Michelle, mom of one
Niantic, Connecticut

You never know, those encounters might result in wonderful friendships. These friendships do have a few strings attached, however. What, exactly, do these relationship need?

Dependability: Sure, even the word *dependability* is at the mercy of your family. Typically kids get into some kind of routine (which may change with the seasons or the school year), so when you feel a schedule settling in, make a standing date.

> My number one training partner was once merely an acquaintance. After seeing each other in a maternity store, we set a date to run together. Since then our children have become good friends and look forward to playdates while we run.
>
> —Laurie

Flexibility: As much as you need a training partner you can count on, and who can count on you, circumstances may arise when you can't meet up as planned. Try to give each other as much warning as possible and see if you can reschedule instead of cancel.

Similar Schedules: One of the most common indicators of having a similar schedule is having similar-aged children or the same work schedule. If you both block out large chunks of your day at the same time, then your "free time" just might coincide.

A Mute Button: If your gab-o-meters go off at the same time then you're probably well matched. If you don't like to talk or don't like to listen to someone go on and on, then Chatty Cathy won't be your ideal sweat mate. Conversation can be a beautiful thing to help pass the time, but sometimes silence *is* golden. Know how to tactfully express your needs.

Enabling Behavior: A friend who shares workouts with you is wonderful. True love is found when that friend helps you get your workout in when you otherwise might not. When your workout becomes as important as her workout, and vice versa, how can you *not* be fit?

Inspiration in the Perspiration

Working out with another woman—particularly another mom—will do wonders for your motivation. If you're struggling to get out the door because you're mom to two kids, a needy mutt, and a pet salamander, it becomes more difficult to offer up excuses for missing your workout when your workout partner has four kids, one with special needs, an ailing mother, and a husband who travels during the week. Sometimes just knowing the effort it takes someone else to squeeze in a workout will inspire you to do the same and validate your dedication to getting or staying in shape.

The more you get to know other fit moms, the more you'll realize you're not alone. You'll hear stories about kids who wouldn't go to bed the night before (yet their mom still makes it to her early morning workout), about babysitters who cancel at the last minute (so Mom pushes the jogger instead), and about spouses who complain about being on kid duty while Mom runs (but she stands her ground and goes anyway).

The small battles waged against you in your quest for fitness are fairly common. You don't need to take comfort in others' struggles, but a little empathy and awe work both ways. Share combat stories and strategies with the right women and you'll find the motivation and support to succeed more often.

Team Therapy

Work past the motivation, spend time with those girlfriends on a regular basis, and you'll discover a network of friends like none other. Perhaps it's the vulnerability we show when pushing our bodies to new limits. Maybe it's that the focus often *appears* to be elsewhere (the next mile, the next pose, the next volley). For whatever reason, women engaged in sport together have a bond that leaves all the "junk" behind. There is no makeup required, no perfect hair needed (though we all know a few women who get pretty before getting sweaty). Push past the surface and we've got so much more to work with. We've got our *real* selves.

And so the talk turns to stuff that matters when it needs to. Exercise can quickly filter out the small talk, common courtesies, and current events when something more pressing is rising to the surface: careers in limbo, faltering marriages, depression, family conflicts. Often what we want from our training pals—just someone to listen to us—we get as we trudge through our neighborhoods or on neighboring treadmills. In our busy lives, when all we typically give our friendships is a quick e-mail, text message, or call from our cell in between soccer games, having the luxury of twenty or thirty minutes, maybe even an hour, to talk face-to-face with someone (even if it is on the move) is rare indeed. Just knowing you have someone to talk to can lighten the load. Sometimes it's as if the talking itself releases a valve on the pressure we feel. Defining the problem helps us understand it better and helps to formulate the solutions to carry on when the exercise is over.

And sometimes when we really don't know what to do and we need an unbiased opinion, our sweaty sisters can step in. Obviously our workout partners can't take the place of a professional therapist, but loving friends who have our best interests at heart may have useful insight—even when that advice is to "see a professional therapist."

When we need encouragement from friends, training partners somehow know and give whatever they can. When we need a good laugh, it's always there. A shoulder to cry on is probably inches away. Sweaty maybe, but sturdy and supportive—a good shoulder nonetheless.

Mixing Sweat with Your Social Life

Sometimes working out with friends is just plain fun—fun disguised as a workout, or maybe a workout disguised as fun. No matter how you look at it, it's what you *want* to do with your would-be alone time. Your girls' night out doesn't have to take place in a smoky bar. Get creative, multitasking mamas! Here are some suggestions for mixing sweat with your social life.

1. Open your existing friendships up to fitness. Suggest something physical for your next girls' night out. Maybe it's your moms' group, your coworkers, or your college friends. Ballroom dancing? A group tennis lesson? Find out what the group has always wanted to do.

2. Plan an adventure-night series with your workout pals. Take turns scheduling activities and sports that are new to the whole group. Hit a rock-climbing gym, take a speed-skating lesson, go orienteering. Reward your efforts with pure social time, too. Organize a cookout or dinner at a restaurant. And it's good to include your families from time to time.

3. Set up a fitness playgroup. What modern mother isn't part of a playgroup or two? Do we all have to sit around and watch our babies play? Take turns heading out for your own play session.

4. Make your book club mobile. If you're part of a book club, suggest that you take your discussion outdoors so you can walk and talk about it. Or, if you're part of a group of walking or running friends, suggest a book that you all can read and discuss at a future workout.

5. Take an active girls' trip. Plan a getaway with a physical goal: a biking trip through fall foliage, a hiking trip out west, or a destination marathon. Prepare for your trip together and the training will be as much fun as the vacation.

The Stink

We said before that this whole girlfriend thing might sound too good to be true. Truth be told, it sometimes is. Depending on your level of fitness and commitment to your sport, you might find that the friendly competitive spirit isn't always so friendly. A number of issues might arise that cause a rift in your relationship. An obvious issue that can arise is jealousy: say, if you meet your weight loss goal and your training pal doesn't, or if a friend's insecurity comes between you when you outgrow the pace of your group.

We'd like to believe that our friends would support our personal victories and feel triumph in them, too (after all, they were part of it in some ways). Sometimes, unfortunately, grown women can't feel joy for you because they're stuck on feeling bad for themselves. Instead of "Wow! I'm really happy for you!" It's "Geez, your success makes me feel incompetent." Of course, she might not come out and say this; it may take the form of more passive-aggressive behavior, such as not showing up for workouts, canceling them, or withdrawing from the friendship. It might take the form of biting comments or "making fun" of your success or—worse—petty gossip.

Check back to chapter 12 for information on what to do when you don't get the support you need. If problems do arise, make sure you handle them with respect.

However, as with any friendship, you want the relationship to be uplifting, not something that drags you down. If you can't work out the problem and if this "friend" continues with her negative, passive-aggressive behavior, then you're better off spending that energy on other friends, new friends, your family, or your own fitness. Perhaps you can use your own positive energy to help support someone else in their fitness success. That's what mentoring, and the next secret, are all about.

MOM **2** MOM

A friend asked me to join a gym with her. Then I started running with her. Now she refuses to run with me. She says I am too fast!

—Grainne, mom of two
Stamford, Connecticut

Secret Number 5

ACT LIKE
OTHERS ARE
WATCHING
BECAUSE THEY ARE

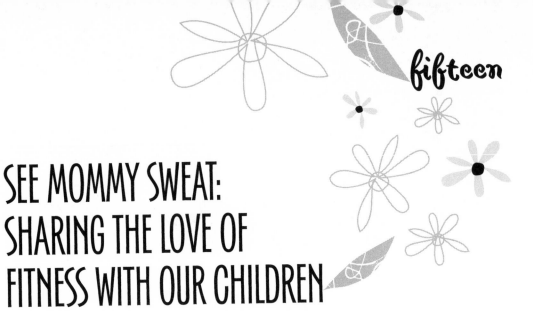

fifteen

SEE MOMMY SWEAT: SHARING THE LOVE OF FITNESS WITH OUR CHILDREN

Have you become your mother yet? If she was a good role model for you then you probably already know this is not necessarily a bad thing. Now that we are mothers ourselves, though, what we experienced as children is less important than what we want our own children to experience. We understand the power that our mere presence has on our kids. We want to make our influence count, and it's clear that our actions speak louder than words.

Throughout this book we've worked hard to help you squash any mother guilt you might feel when you take a little "me time" to squeeze in a workout. And while we think doing something good for yourself can stand on its own merit, you can also take satisfaction in knowing that when you work out you are engaging in good behavior that your child is likely to engage in as well. And what parent wouldn't want their child to grow up fit and active?

Yet it's not enough to drop the kids off at Little League. If you want to ensure your kids embody a fit lifestyle, they need to grow up in a home where fitness is a family value. If Mom (and let's hope Dad)

MOM 2 MOM

I think as parents we have a duty to be a good example for our children. Not only are we teaching them it's important to be healthy and take care of your body, we are also showing them to love themselves and to have self-respect and goals.

—Melissa, mom of three
Turlock, California

is active, then odds are much better that kids will mirror that behavior and make fitness a habit when they're adults. (And you thought you were working up a sweat to justify those Oreo Double Stuf cookies!)

It makes sense that fitness should be a part of parenting. As mothers we are guardians of our children's health. We assume this role willingly, even unconsciously, as part of our maternal instinct. Obviously the younger our children, the more we exert this influence: taking them to the doctor, feeding them healthful foods, assuring they get enough sleep, protecting them from harm. As they grow, so do their independence and the choices they make about their health. For instance, we may give them money for the vending machine at school, but we can't make the selection for them. We can only hope that we've established a pattern of healthy eating at home that they want to continue to emulate on their own.

But don't despair if your kid picks junk food every time. They tend to follow similar patterns as their parents, eventually, so it's best not to cram it down their throats. You know how easily this can backfire. If you want it too badly for them, they might become the couch potato, slacker kid out of spite. So remember what we said earlier about attracting versus repelling. Same goes with our children.

Show, Don't Tell

Being a fitness role model for your children can start very young, before they are likely to join you for workouts. This doesn't make getting a workout in with children around any easier. Think two-year-old with an attachment disorder: As troublesome as it is to peel said child off your leg to go do your fit thing, and as futile as explanations and negotiations are at this age, start telling them why you go. Explain why Mommy needs to go walk with her friends or ride her bike or play tennis or go to yoga class. "Mommy needs to exercise because it makes her feel better so we can have more fun later." Keep it simple, but make your point. Then when you return, make sure they see you happy. *Really* happy. Even if you're not that happy, a little exaggeration will help drive that point home. And then at other times in your day (when you're not threatening to leave) talk about "when Mommy goes to exercise," so they see it as a positive in your life. Eventually they may see it as a positive in theirs, as well.

But we know we can't be fitness Pollyannas all the time. As your children get a little older, it's important for them to understand that, while most of the time you love exercise (come on, don't you love it just a little bit?) and want to do it, sometimes you don't. On those days you don't feel like heading out the door to sweat, you can share that with them, too, but let them know you do it anyway because it's good for you (like eating whatever vegetable they find distasteful).

If you've come to fitness late, don't despair. You can have these same conversations with older kids. In fact, you may not have to do much talking at all. Showing, not telling, can be more powerful, especially with teenagers. They will see the transformative power exercise has on you. They know what it feels like to have a happy mom in the house.

A few years ago I asked my daughters what they'd rather do: watch a movie or go to the gym. The only reason I gave them the option is because I was *sure* they would pick the movie. I had already run that morning but had mentally penciled in a yoga class for the afternoon. However, after spending all day at a friend's house, lounging in perfect sunny weather, swimming in the lake, and eating yummy food, I was sun drunk and ready to go home. Watching a movie with my eyes closed in our dark basement seemed a nice way to cap off our day. So imagine my surprise when the girls sang out unanimously, "Go to the gym!"

—Kara

What Kids Have to Say About Mom's Fitness

"I like when you exercise so we can get more time to play."
—*Stuart, six*

"You encourage the whole family to work out and look, we're all ripped!"
—*Sam, eight*

"It's pretty good because it makes you more fit and even makes you taller."
—*Sophie, eight*

"I like the Y. We get M&M's."
—*Ben, three*

"I love it when you go work out, because then we get
Daddy and he lets us watch a movie and eat popcorn."
—*Isabella Grace, four*

"I think it's beautiful because when you run it makes me want to run."
—*Kezia, eight*

"It's good that you get a lot of exercise because
your muscles get stronger and help you grow."
—*Harry, eight*

Learning to Love Fitness

We are born to love fitness. It's in our blood. If you need proof, just watch an infant laugh as she learns to kick her legs in the crib or bat at those tempting toys we hang from their car seats. Toddlers run in circles, screaming joyfully at the top of their lungs—deafening but convincing evidence that most of us delight in physical activity from a very early age.

Perhaps our role as parents isn't so much to teach our children how to be fit, but rather to ensure this inborn love affair with activity is not lost—that our children grow up valuing the attitude and behavior with which they were born. So at a very early age, it's important to let kids be kids, so to speak. Let them gravitate toward activity and experience fitness as creative play.

As your children develop the coordination necessary for organized or solo sports, take time to teach them the fundamentals in a playful, safe environment. These are the elements of Sports 101 and they are just as important as learning the ABCs. The building blocks of sports include important things such as how to throw overhand, which is important in many sports, from baseball, softball, and football to less obvious pursuits such as tennis and volleyball. You want to encourage your children to learn basic athletic skills in a fun and relaxed atmosphere. Easy enough, right? And yet we still say people "throw like a girl," which really means they have never been taught how to correctly throw a ball. It's our responsibility to teach our children the basics—running and jumping, throwing and kicking a ball. If you're not sure how to do that, stick around for Little League practice. Yes, we've encouraged you to use your kids' sports

> My uncle Bob, who was a baseball coach, tried to teach all of us girls how to throw and hit a baseball. But I was never comfortable with the "ball sports" growing up and assumed I was not any good at them, mostly because I didn't try or was afraid to try. I want to make sure my girls don't grow up with that same reluctance.
>
> —Kara

practices for your own workout, but this is one of those times it might make sense to stay and learn proper technique yourself. That way you can practice with your child at home without too much trouble.

It's best to teach kids those fundamental skills without the added baggage of competition. In this environment they focus their success on their personal development rather than winning or losing a game. After all, we want our children to enjoy activity for the sake of movement and healthy living. So head out to the backyard and don't worry about the score.

Parenting is less about "raising" children as it is allowing them to become who they are meant to be. Take note of the activities that give them the most pleasure and the ones they excel at. Guide them into finding the activities that are true expressions of themselves, just like you're doing for yourself. With any luck, it might be the same, and you and your children can stay fit together for years to come.

Family Fitness

We're convinced that a family that sweats together, gets closer together. There is something wonderful about sharing sweaty moments with others. We discussed how quickly friendships can turn intimate over a little sweat in the last chapter. It's the same theory with you and your family. Getting fit with your children will provide you with a number of opportunities to discuss some of the deeper things in life, such as the importance of hard work, how to overcome challenges, and how to deal with success and failure.

To develop your identity as a fit family, there are a number of things you can do:

1. Make it fun for everyone—especially if you have young children. Do what you can to make your kids love sports by providing a fun outlet for them to get physical. Consider obstacle courses, lawn sports, yard games, and scavenger hunts to get little legs moving. Geocaching is a popular way for families to get outside and explore. Using GPS coordinates, geocachers take and leave items from hidden caches they find in parks and on public lands across the country. See http://www.geocaching.com/ for more information.

2. If you're looking for more structured sports, find something everyone can participate in at his or her own level. Sports such as martial arts and rock climbing are appropriate for all ages. A trip to the local beach for a lake swim or an all-comers track meet works well, too. Sure, everyone's skill levels will be slightly different, but sharing the passion for a particular sport or activity will bring everyone together. Better that than a television show, right?

3. Set a family goal. Train for a local 5K walk or family fun event. Join a family softball league or plan to ride your bikes a set distance for which you will all train. It doesn't need to be a public event, but at some point an event can do wonders for everyone's enthusiasm. Take the time to make T-shirts for the family to promote your own "team." Reward the family with a celebration when you reach your goal.

4. Set individual goals and support one another. Give everyone (including Mom and Dad) the opportunity to set goals and compete while the rest of the family watches and cheers from the sidelines. This can be in the form of a soccer game, volleyball match, or bicycle race. The important part is having the family members there to support one another.

5. Cheer others on as spectators. Take the kids to local events. This doesn't have to be in the form of professional athletics; head to the local high school or a nearby college to watch the competition. Get your kids cheering and make it fun.

6. Volunteer at an event. Take time as a family to support a local, national, or global health and fitness organization. Donate your time at a local fun run by volunteering

at a water stop. Get the whole family there and support your athletic community together.

7. Reward your children. This variation on the "chore chart" isn't nearly as hard to keep going. Fill in sports or activities your kids enjoy and encourage them to earn stars by keeping active. When your daughter turns off the television and heads outside to play soccer without being asked, give her two stars. Simply rewarding positive, healthy choices encourages kids to continue making good decisions.

Got Daughters?

Most young kids—regardless of gender—love running, playing catch, and just being active in general. But unlike their male classmates, a high percentage of adolescent girls quit sports in the junior high school years.

While social pressure has something to do with this, childhood experiences also play a role. Providing our children with a positive foundation in athletics and supporting and encouraging their pursuits make sports a welcoming territory for them. Having confidence in their bodies' abilities will help them get past the most difficult years for sports—between ages twelve and sixteen.

Perhaps more important than raising fit daughters is raising safe daughters. Statistics show that girls who participate in sports have lower rates of alcohol and drug abuse, and are less likely to smoke, get pregnant, or drop out of school.

Experts suggest that, besides being good role models for our daughters and teaching them the basic skills necessary for sports, we should introduce young girls to sports in mixed-

MOM 2 MOM

I love it that my daughters see me working out and see that I surround myself with healthy, powerful women. My daughters think that's the norm and that exercising is a part of everyday life.

—Kuay, mom of two
Coppell, Texas

I once took my oldest to our babysitter's high school track meet. What a great move! My daughter loved meeting all of the teenage girls, and our babysitter felt supported and excited to show off her little friend. Years later, that babysitter is a good family friend, someone I know we'll stay in touch with for years to come.

—Laurie

gender groups. Find coed teams—T-ball, soccer, hockey, basketball. This will help teach the importance of sports and fitness as a gender-neutral pursuit—particularly helpful to developing our female athletes.

Also, don't limit your sports-as-entertainment outings to men-only events. Take your kids to see women's high school, collegiate, and professional athletic events, too.

Of course, it's unclear if sports attract high-achieving, highly functional young women, or if athletics foster those behaviors. In the end, what matters is that our daughters are doing things that help them stay away from risky behaviors. The good news is that these benefits kick in most effectively during early adolescence when girls are most at risk. The key is to get your daughter started in sports early on.

We know our kids are watching—one another, their parents, the world around them. With so much we can't control, it makes sense to be certain that the messages we send our kids are positive and healthy. Modeling a fit life is another contribution we make to their future while taking care of our own. Need more ideas to engage kids in fitness? The next chapter is all about ways to work out with your kids, no matter what age they are.

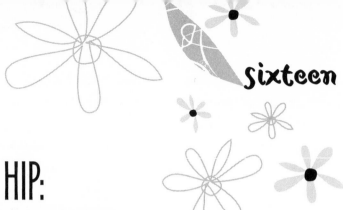

sixteen

JOINED AT THE HIP: EXERCISE STRATEGIES FOR BABIES AND TODDLERS

Back in chapter 3 we outlined the four ways moms with young children can create time for fitness: make time, take time, snare time, or share time. Accomplishing a workout is relatively easy when you make time or take time because it's just you and your workout; you delegate child care to someone else. Exercise with your children alongside you can be a bit more challenging. But for many moms, "sharing time" is the best option for exercise, especially if they work a full-time job outside the home and have limited time with their kids, or for single moms who can't tag-team child care with their partner, or moms who have a toddler with severe attachment issues. Whenever you find yourself in an exercise stalemate, it might seem easier to throw up your hands and surrender your fit life. Not so fast.

Even if you do have ample time during your day to exercise without your children, you might consider

MOM 2 MOM

When my girls were little I put them in a double jogging stroller with plenty of snacks. We would jog to the library, get a bunch of books, go to the park where there is a running trail, and run while my girls looked at their new books. Then we would stop at the playground before running the long way home. We would sing "I think I can, I think I can" from *The Little Engine That Could* running up the hill by our house. My girls are now eighteen and sixteen and they still remember those early days.

—Michele, mom of two
Coppell, Texas

letting them join you every now and then to establish a pattern of family fitness. Witnessing you in the act of exercise reinforces your kids' understanding that fitness is important and fun and that fitness belongs in their world, too.

As you experience these unique exercise moments and share time exercising with your children, remember that your goal is twofold: to accomplish your own workout and to expose your children to exercise. Even if the workout isn't exactly what you had hoped for in terms of calorie burn or intensity, you are still making fine use of your time.

In this chapter we'll tackle exercise options for moms with young or dependent children, when oftentimes, like it or not, we're bringing them along for the ride. In the next chapter we'll offer suggestions for getting older kids to join in the fun.

Fitness with a Newborn

The first step in any postpartum fitness plan is the same for everyone: Get the OK from your doctor or midwife. While one woman may be comfortable returning to exercise one or two weeks after birth, it may take months before another woman is ready. Listen to your body and remember that sleep takes precedence over exercise at this stage. Your body is healing and does its best repair work while you're sleeping. Above all, nurture yourself. You've asked a lot of your body during the last nine months, so do only those things that feel good to you. That said, there are suitable ways to return to fitness with a newborn, and even exercises you *should* do.

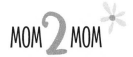

MOM 2 MOM

I have been nursing or pregnant (or both) for almost four years now. Sometimes my body just feels too tired to exercise!

—Stephanie, mom of two
Pleasant View, Tennessee

Build Pelvic-Floor Strength

No matter how you gave birth to your child, carrying a baby to term puts an undue burden on the pelvic-floor muscles, which can ultimately lead to bladder-control problems. Heck, even if you adopted, every woman can benefit from a little work on the pelvic floor.

While a lot of new moms are tempted to resume their prepregnancy exercise status as soon as possible, unless you first rebuild pelvic-floor strength, you are inviting trouble to the rest of your body. The pelvic floor is the very bottom of your core. You know you need a strong core to prevent injury and maximize your strength. Regardless of whether or not you're raring to work up a sweat, you'll need a strong bottom core as your baby gets heavier and you lift and hold this growing bundle of joy. Fitness should begin at this bottom core—your pelvic floor—and radiate upward and outward.

We can't talk about the pelvic floor without talking about Kegels, that "down-there" exercise everyone says you're supposed to do and do often. You've probably convinced yourself that you're the only one who doesn't do enough of them. If so, we promise to make you feel better about this.

Just in case you've been living under a rock, a Kegel is the concentrated version of the same muscle contraction that stops your urine stream (or squeezes a wayward tampon or prevents you from passing gas during yoga class). Stopping urine is something that may not come so easily after having a baby, especially, say, when you sneeze or have a coughing attack.

> **I think of Kegels as a fun little secret. It's kind of like wearing no underwear.**
>
> —Laurie

A correctly executed Kegel shouldn't be a forceful gripping of the muscles, however, but rather a gentle sustained squeeze followed by a complete release. Think elevator rising to the second floor. Try it ten times, holding for a few seconds to make sure you can, and then release.

The releasing step is one many women leave out. Biomechanical scientist Katy Bowman reminds us that a tight muscle does not equate to a strong muscle. A muscle must be in its optimal position—not too tight, not too loose—to function at its best. So after a Kegel, be sure to release all the way to the point you feel you could pee.

In the first few weeks after delivery, Kegels should be part of your postpartum recovery. Pick something as a prompt, perhaps nursing or bottle-feeding your baby or changing diapers to help you remember to Kegel several times a day.

Rather than tell you to do hundreds of Kegels a day every day ad infinitum, we're going against the grain to say: Don't go overboard with the Kegels. Yes, contrary to popular opinion, which suggests hundreds of Kegels are necessary to repair the pelvic floor, the Kegel, like anything in life, can be too much of a good thing. Here's why: After childbirth the goal is to turn the pelvic floor from a drooping hammock into a taut trampoline. A Kegel overdose, according to Bowman, can make the pelvic floor muscles too tight (especially if you're not training that muscle to release after each contraction). This can further compromise pelvic-floor strength because these tight muscles can tug too much on the attached bony structures, throwing your pelvis out of alignment, thereby preventing the pelvic floor from distributing the weight of your internal organs evenly. If you've ever experienced pain in your pubic bone or tail bone, you know what we're talking about here. And suddenly you're back to peeing with every sneeze again.

Bowman, who is also the director of the Restorative Exercise Institute and creator of the *Aligned and Well* DVD series, suggests new moms engage the muscles that connect to the pelvic floor—the gluteal muscles, the inner thighs, and the hips—and keep these muscles supple by stretching. She says a telltale sign that a woman's gluteal muscles aren't pulling their weight is the flat "mom butt." You know what we're talking about. It's not pretty, especially in "mom jeans."

There is one move in particular that fights "mom butt" and the pelvic floor weakness it creates: a deep squat. This is the kind of squat you see toddlers assume all the time: to poop, to pick up a dead bug, to play with toys on the floor. So make like a toddler and squat whenever you can: for instance, when you pick up your baby from the car seat or sit next to the tub as you bathe your baby. Bowman says squatting will lengthen and strengthen the butt muscles, hamstrings, quadriceps, calves, and psoas muscles (the front of your hips). Very few exercises can do all that. In fact, she suggests this is the best position to Kegel in, for optimal and long-term pelvic-floor strength. You can find more information at http://www.restorativeexercise.com.

While you're rebuilding your core you might want to knit together that reservoir that is separating your abdominal muscles—also referred to as diastasis recti. Throwing yourself into sit-ups and crunches will not put your abs together and, worse still, will put undue pressure on the pelvic floor. Physical therapist Shirley Sahrmann, who specializes in abdominal rehabilitation, developed a series of five progressive exercises to reengage the pelvic-floor and core muscles during and after pregnancy, which we've adapted from the book *Prenatal and Postpartum Exercise Design* by Gwen Hyatt, MS, and Catherine Cram, MS. You must be able to do one before going on to the next. If you are pregnant, perform these exercises while supported by your elbows. If you've recently delivered a baby, wait until any incisions or tearing has healed.

Basic breath. This step helps you isolate the correct abdominal muscles. Lie on your back, arms at your side with your knees bent, feet flat on the floor. Take a deep breath and on the exhale, pull your belly button toward your spine, concentrating on the muscles below your belly button. Contract the muscles without flattening your back or tilting your pelvis. Keep the natural curve in your back. Relax and inhale. When you are able to contract the muscles below your belly button without arching or flattening your back, you can move on to the exercises.

> Sahrmann exercises were my main workout, along with walking, for the first three months after my fourth child was born. The rift down my abdomen closed up fairly quickly.
>
> —Kara

1. Lying on your back, arms at your side with your knees bent and feet flat on the floor, perform the basic breath. Keep one knee bent, and slowly slide the other leg out along the floor until it is fully extended. Then slide the leg back into position and relax. Alternate legs. Begin with one to five repetitions with each leg, maintaining the correct abdominal contraction and keeping the natural curve in your back. Gradually work your way up to twenty repetitions before moving on to the second exercise.

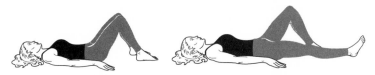

2. Set up the same as number one. Perform the basic breath. Raise one knee toward your chest and slowly straighten it out so that it is parallel to, but not touching, the floor. Return that leg to the starting position and relax. Alternate legs. Once you have gradually worked your way up to twenty repetitions without losing the abdominal contraction, progress to the next exercise.

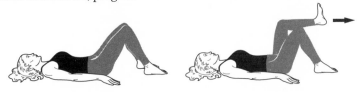

3. Lie on your back with your knees bent. As you perform the basic breath, slowly lift your knees toward your body so they are up at a ninety-degree angle. Keep one leg up, while dropping the remaining bent leg to touch the floor with your foot. Raise it back up. Alternate legs. You might be able to start with only a few repetitions per leg while holding the abdominal contraction, but once you've worked up to twenty repetitions you may add on the next exercise.

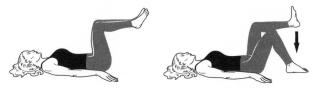

4. Set up the same as number 3, with knees lifted and bent at a ninety-degree angle while you perform the basic breath. Slowly extend one leg out so that it is parallel to, but not touching, the floor. Bring the leg back to a ninety-degree angle, and repeat on the other leg, working up to ten repetitions per leg. With each repetition, employ the basic breath and hold the abdominal contraction until the leg is straightened, without compromising the low back. If the back arches you should not progress. Once you are strong enough to finish twenty repetitions, move on to the fifth exercise.

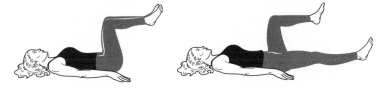

5. Lying on your back with your legs extended perform the basic breath and bring both legs straight up one at a time. Your legs should be at a ninety-degree angle at the hips. Slowly lower both legs together toward the floor. Go only as far as you feel is comfortable, or to the point where the back starts to arch. Return to the start and repeat, going only as far as you can go without the back arching, eventually aiming to go parallel to the floor. Work up to ten. In time aim for twenty.

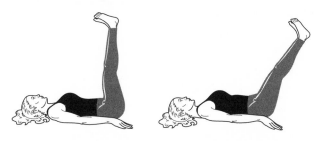

While these exercises can give you something to focus on during those first postpartum months, keep them in your exercise regimen as your children grow. (In fact, you don't even have to have given birth to benefit from them.)

Yoga/Pilates Baby

If you practiced yoga or Pilates before or during pregnancy, then you know they are both soothing to the body and vital to rebuilding lost core strength. You may find "baby and me" classes, but consider buying a video or two, or renting them from your local library, for use at home. These workouts are easy to pause for a bit when you need to nurse, change a poopy diaper, or sooth a colicky newborn. Just continue where you left off.

Bounce

You may already be familiar with the "birthing" ball, which many women use to find comfort during labor. It's the same physio ball you see at the gym for workouts. If you don't already have one in your home, consider adding this valuable piece of equipment, and even replacing your rocking chair with it. Bouncing on the ball is great for your core, and babies love it. It is our cure for colic and core malaise. This is motherhood multitasking at its best. Try these variations while you're at it. Keep your core tight, stay in control, and move deliberately.

> One of my twins, a sensory-seeking kid from the start, could only be lulled to sleep by big bounces on the ball. Often, a the same time, I used one foot to rock the other twin in a bouncy seat on the floor. That was my postpartum "core"-dination challenge test.
>
> —Kara

- Bounce while rocking your pelvis side to side, then front to back.
- Bounce while holding one foot slightly off the floor (not too high—remember, you're holding a baby!).
- Bounce while alternately placing a heel on the floor.

If your baby doesn't need to bounce, try these exercises while keeping the ball as still as possible.

Baby Steps

Most women are ready to walk and get fresh air relatively soon after birth (oh, to walk without all that extra weight!). Even wearing baby in a carrier is far more comfortable than the nine-month waddle. If you've had a surgical birth you may need more recovery time and should start by pushing your baby in a stroller before wearing the little one. Start with a walk to the mailbox. Gradually move up to ten, fifteen, then twenty minutes. Before you know it, you and baby will be best of power-walking partners.

Fitness with an Infant

"Work out while the baby takes a nap." It can be such moronic advice. On the one hand it seems too obvious to mention; on the other it seems futile because napping can be so darn unpredictable. In fact, "unpredictable" sums up life with an infant. You never know whether you're going to get the angel baby who coos and smiles all day, sleeps on cue, and naps so long you freak out and begin to check for breathing, or the baby who poops up the back of her diaper, is incessantly hungry, and refuses to be put down. And strangely we could be describing the same baby on different days, perhaps the same day. The only way to make a workout happen is to be as unpredictable as your infant, which means having many options from which to choose.

> When our first daughter was young and still taking regular naps, my husband and I would plan our runs around naptime. She became such a predictable sleeper that we once put in over twenty miles with her sleeping in the jogger. She started out sleepy, eventually fell asleep, and woke up just blocks from home, well rested. Now in grade school, she'd never sit still that long. She can't make it twenty miles, but she's right out there alongside us on her bike for shorter runs.
>
> —Laurie

Work Out When Baby Naps

Yes, we said it was moronic advice, but we still have to suggest it, right? Hopefully that means we're eternal optimists, instead of morons. We know this won't work for you all the time, so keep your expectations low. Pop in your favorite exercise video, tune into the FitTV channel, log onto your favorite workout Web site, or start up your treadmill or other home-exercise option. Sometimes you might get to finish a whole workout *and* take a shower; other times you might not get ten minutes to sweat. Be happy with whatever time you get and try again tomorrow.

More Baby Steps

Walking, running, or cycling with your baby in tow will get your heart rate going. It's also a wonderful way to let your baby enjoy nature and the fresh air along with you. For the baby who doesn't nap, it can be the perfect antidote.

Make sure your baby is big enough to be safely strapped into the stroller or trailer and heed the advice of manufacturers and your doctor. Generally speaking, your baby should have sufficient neck strength to keep her head up during the ride. Some have special slings for infants or adaptors that allow you to snap your car carrier directly inside.

Consider the following checklist (stash the items in the handy pocket of the stroller) to avoid a quick return:

1. Sunglasses. Most babies don't like them, but they can be carefully placed on the unsuspecting once asleep.

2. Hat. Another easily placed sun shield, even better for keeping sun off baby's delicate skin.

3. Diapers and wipes. Definitely change your baby before you leave, but keep a stash just in case. Sometimes a clean diaper can make the difference between contentment and tears.

4. Comfort item. Whatever your baby uses to self-soothe, bring it along. Pacifiers, teething rings, your toothbrush—have it handy. If your baby takes a bottle or sippy cup and can hold it up himself, take one along, too. If you bring your child's favorite lovey, consider securing it to the stroller or their clothes. If accidentally thrown overboard, you may grieve the loss more than your child.

When our daughter lost her beloved Dirty Dolly on a long run with my husband, we combed his run course for over an hour. We eventually found Dirty perched atop a sign along the lake. It really is about karma. I do the same thing for other parents now.

—Laurie

5. Blanket. No doubt your body temperature will go up during your run. But cruising along with the breeze created by even a brisk walk will make baby's temperature much different from your own. Be prepared but don't overdo it. Take the smallest blanket that will work or you'll be making frequent stops to gather and tuck.

6. Weather shield. Most strollers and bike trailers come with sun canopies. Be sure to find one with the best coverage possible. It's also a good idea to look for a stroller or trailer that has (usually at an additional cost) an optional weather shield. A good low-cost option is to carry along a waterproof crib pad. Throw this over the top of the stroller and voilà! baby stays dry. Either option is a great method to protect baby from cold and rain and, if you are from a colder clime, will extend your "tandem" running sessions later into the year.

Baby Entertainment

When your baby wakes up from a nap and you're not quite done jogging on your treadmill or exercising to a video, plop her down beside you and let her watch. She may think you're the most thrilling thing ever. Especially if you integrate one or all of the following to entertain her:

1. Let baby move, too. Sit your little one inside a stroller, swing, or jump seat while you're working out. Then, use these mobile forms of restraint to your advantage by giving your baby a push or swing at unexpected intervals. Add in a crazy giggle and you're golden.

2. Dress the part. Got a crazy T-shirt you've been hiding away for the past ten years? Maybe an old Tweety Bird or Elmo shirt from the days of old? Now is the time to don your crazy apparel. Consider anything that might mesmerize or entertain.

3. Get your baby groove on. We all love to work out to our favorite tunes, but, like it or not, now is the time to rock to *Yo Gabba Gabba!*, *Sesame Street*, Raffi, or whatever engages your child.

4. Accessorize. Baby toys are great decorations for exercise equipment. Find toys with Velcro and secure them to your handlebars or the frame of your treadmill. Heck, with a little string, toys fit nicely on almost anything—even a yogi-mom's feet.

Fitness with a Toddler

Having a toddler makes family fitness infinitely more interesting. Toddlers have opinions. Toddlers know exactly what they want to do. More often than not, this is not what you want to do. If you haven't already learned the benefits of deep breathing, now is the time. That said, when your plans and those of your toddler happen to coincide, the group workout is a wondrous motherhood-affirming moment.

Roll Along

The best part about a jogging stroller or bike trailer is that the toddler is strapped in. OK, we should be nicer to the toddlers. They are more loving, hilarious, and cuter than they are maddening. Even if they initially refuse to go along for the ride, once they get going, they're usually happy. You can help engage them by searching out favorite objects (school buses, dump trucks, puppies, and the like) and singing their favorite songs. If you really want to win them over, stop at a favorite park.

Your checklist for running with a toddler includes everything we mention above for running with an infant, along with the following:

1. Toys/books. Bring a few toys, but nothing so small that you won't notice when your toddler launches it from the stroller. Consider attaching your child's favorite stuffed animal, doll, or blanket to the stroller with Velcro, a safety pin, or duct tape. Unless you want to double your distance, retracing your steps to find a much-loved toy can be frustrating. Even worse is not discovering the special toy is missing until bedtime, when you *really* need it.

MOM 2 MOM

My two-year-old hated riding along on my bike with me, so in an effort to soothe his fears and wrestle him into the seat, I let him bring two favorite stuffed animals along the first time out. I talked to him the whole ride, but I couldn't see how he was doing. When I got back, I realized he had fallen asleep, and the stuffed animals were nowhere to be found. He woke up and shrieked, "my fwiends!" So we headed back out to rescue them. The rescue was a success, I got in twice as much biking as I had planned, and I learned a valuable lesson!

—Julie, mom of two
Billings, Montana

Talking games are great for keeping my recovery workouts easy. If I'm talking, I can't push myself as hard.

—Laurie

2. Snacks. Nothing sloppy here. Make them easy-to-grab items cut into small pieces so it takes them longer to eat. Raisins and crackers work well.

3. Water bottle. Something just like Mom's. Who knew a water bottle could be both functional and entertaining!

4. Notebook and a few crayons. With these in hand, your options are endless. Pick up leaves and sticks along the way and let the kids decorate. Anything goes.

5. Games. Put together a list of games you can play together as you run, walk, or stroll. Scavenger hunts and games of "I Spy" are at the top of our list.

MOM 2 MOM

My son loves his push-along car (with a handle). I amazingly find this much easier to push than a jogging stroller. It just glides across the pavement. My son absolutely loves it. It is a bit loud and people look, but they always smile at him because he is having a great time! And so am I. I can push him up to an hour and get six miles in. And, he thinks we are just playing and "driving" around the neighborhood!

—Jamie, mom of two
Sun Prairie, Wisconsin

Playroom Fitness

Sometimes, just being in the same room together is enough to placate a toddler. Try moving along to your favorite exercise video and ask your child to exercise "with" you. (A hippity hop ball makes a great child-size version of a physio ball.) If you need a cardio workout, turn on your favorite tunes (or theirs) and have a dance party. Sometimes you can use your toddler as a fitness prop: Have them "ride" on your back for push-ups or sit on your abs for pelvic raises. Get creative; they'll think you're better than a theme park.

I admit, exercise with my kids is usually Plan B. I prefer the ease and freedom of working out on my own. What I've discovered in those times when I do acquire a successful workout in the company of children is that I glean a whole new layer of satisfaction from it. Yep, makes me feel like a badass mama.

—Kara

Bedtime Exercises

Even kids with the best bedtime routines often go through a phase of resisting sleep. Sometimes you'll do whatever it takes to get your toddler to sleep—even if that means lying down on the floor next to their crib to coerce them to just close their eyes already. Don't just sit there singing lullabies in the dark. Sing while you move through a series of Sahrmann exercises or your Pilates routine. Do a few crunches or hold that plank for a minute or two. Build on the number of push-ups you can do. Read another story as you stretch. As you're leaning over the crib willing your child to sleep, throw in a set of calf raises.

These early years with young children are some of the most challenging and rewarding as mothers. There are many parenting skills to master, and we believe fitness with children is one of them.

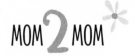

Sometimes we do yoga at bedtime to help my kids settle down.

—Kayris, mom of two
Baltimore, Maryland

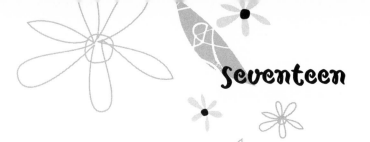

CHILD'S PLAY: EXERCISE STRATEGIES FOR OLDER KIDS AND CHILDREN WITH SPECIAL NEEDS

Just when you've become resigned to a life of diapers and sippy cups, children do the darndest thing: They gain more independence than you are prepared to give. They don't need you as much. As you both adjust to your new freedom, there is a need to reinvent ways to spend time together.

Fitness with School-Age Children

Trying to work in fitness with a toddler will make you second-guess your fitness goals (and your sanity), but before you have the opportunity to snap . . . they grow up a little—just enough to bring some ease into your daily activities. Not only will you experience fewer power struggles (we said fewer, as in fewer than a toddler's), but you'll notice an eagerness to emulate you—even, dare we say, "cooperate."

Roll Along, Part 2

Don't sweat it when your kids outgrow the baby jogger. Chances are they're now riding bikes, scooters, or inline skates. Let them roll alongside you as you walk or run, or go on a bike ride. When selecting your route, consider the following suggestions:

1. Pick a familiar route with a smooth surface so your kids aren't dodging debris and potholes along the way.

2. Look for dedicated bike paths or roads with extra-wide shoulders. Keep your kids between you and the curb on both.

3. Hit routes with water fountains and parks so you can take comfortable breaks whenever needed.

4. Bring along a patch kit and know how to use it. There is nothing worse than ending your workout with a long walk home while carrying a bike.

5. Remember, helmets are not optional for your kids or for you.

Going on a family walk can become more exciting, too, when you run drills to the street corners or various driveways. Mix in some skipping, hopping, or other calisthenics such as jumping jacks and push-ups. Kids love to show you what they've learned in school, so make sure you keep asking what games and skills they are learning in gym class.

Does it snow where you live? Use a dog leash or rope to attach a sled around your waist and pull your kids through the neighborhood. Your neighbors will probably be just as impressed as your children (that is, you will become one of those "super moms" in their eyes). Sledding burns an amazing amount of

MOM 2 MOM

My ten-year-old daughter and I do open-water swims in the summer together. We show up as the sun is rising. I do my workout as she's waiting on shore. Then, she and I go out together and swim side by side. It reminds me of a mama whale and a baby whale swimming. Just as she gets tired, I give her a little push and she starts her stroke again. When we finish, we stand on shore and look at the lake and comment on how fun it was. Those are special moments.

—Kuay, mom of two
Coppell, Texas

calories, especially if you offer to run the sled up the hill each time.

Practice

Odds are good your child is beginning to participate in organized sports. Work on new skills—and get moving—by showing him how it's done. As you practice, focus more on what he's doing right and encourage every step of the way.

Join the Fun

Take your kids to a skating rink, but don't sit there and watch—skate with them. This applies to other activities as well. Try taking a ski or snowboard lesson together or go to a rock-climbing gym. If your children take dance lessons, or tae kwan do, find out if there are simultaneous lessons for adults. If you run, look for events that have kids' events as well. There's nothing like sharing in the accomplishment of running a race.

Play to Win

Some kids are motivated by games and a little friendly competition. Keeping score—in the name of fun—is a way to engage the family together. Have a hula hoop, pogo stick, or jump rope endurance contest. Set up an obstacle course or run drills. Even a game of tag will provide an aerobic workout that would rival any group fitness class.

Fitness with Tweens and Teens

Remember those tiny little newborn toes? Those toes you kissed and cherished are now steaming up oversized sneakers that you don't allow in the house. That toddler that you sometimes wanted to hide from is now a teenager who probably has those same thoughts about you. You know

MOM 2 MOM

We set up obstacle courses at the park and we time one another going through them. My husband and I also pretend we are kids and play on all of the park equipment with the kids while playing tag through it. This is a great workout and bonding experience.

—Melissa, mom of three
Turlock, California

MOM 2 MOM

My children are preteens and running is our favorite family workout. I love that my all-too-often moody teens will open up and talk about what is going on in their lives as we head down the trail.

—Paige, mom of two
Marietta, Georgia

how close you can become with the people you train with: You tend to open up as you sweat, sharing your joys and concerns, connecting in important ways. Sounds like something you'd want to do with your tween or teenager, doesn't it?

Children as Training Partners

If your t(w)een isn't active, you may or may not have success encouraging them to join you in your favorite fitness routine (but keep trying). What's important is to find out what they want to do for physical activity and join them in their pursuit. You may not have ever planned on snowboarding or rock climbing, but you now have a whole new motivation to try. However, if your children are active or want to be active, be prepared. Kids at this age have the potential to be phenomenal athletes.

Play in the Yard

Physical activity doesn't have to be a strain on your time. It doesn't require a whole lot of planning or any cash outlay. Play Frisbee or catch; set up a game of basketball, softball, or volleyball. Things to remember:

1. Be spontaneous. When the basketball game starts going downhill, it's up to you to be enthusiastic about trying something new.

2. Be easygoing. Since friendships are so important, your child's interest may depend on who is (or isn't) watching. So if that "cool kid" from down the street cruises by on her bike, don't be surprised if your son or daughter is suddenly not interested in playing

catch anymore. Don't push the issue; you'll be cool again soon enough.

3. Be inviting. Extend the invitation to your kids' friends. By offering a quick invite, you might get them all involved and interested in continuing their fitness as a team.

4. Be cautious. Use this time together to focus on the positive. Now might not be the best time to bring up that low grade or a breached curfew. If you're trying to develop a fitness bond, then focus on fitness.

5. Be grateful. Let your kids know how much you value time spent together in such a positive way.

Train for an Event

The "event" doesn't have to be a competition (but it could—a local 10K, bike rally, or triathlon); it could be training for that family ski vacation or summer hiking destination. Put a goal out there, prepare a training plan, and conquer it as a family. Many races now have team and/or relay divisions. Train together and compete as a team to celebrate the hard work.

Fitness with Special Needs Children

All you have to do is watch a Special Olympics or Paralympics event to know a disability won't keep a child from pursuing fitness. By making fitness a

MOM 2 MOM

My youngest, Lucy, is ten years old. She has spina bifida and cerebral palsy and uses a wheelchair. Lucy is four feet two inches tall and weighs fifty pounds. Just a few years ago I was almost forty pounds heavier. It was difficult for me to lift and transfer Lucy. I dreaded loading her wheelchair in and out of my car. Around that time my husband, Aaron, hurt his back and the brunt of lifting Lucy now was up to me. Through that experience Aaron and I realized that Lucy's experience of herself and her life was up to us. We could let our experiences end when the pavement ended . . . or we could transform ourselves and all of our lives by becoming strong enough to take Lucy places none of us dared to dream. And Lucy knows the difference. She no longer feels like she is slipping, slipping, slipping as I hurry to move her from her wheelchair to her bed. She has more confidence in me as I lift her out of the tub. She may be slippery, but she knows I really do have her. She has told me, "Mom, I can tell you are stronger."

—Rachel, mom of two
Salt Lake City, Utah

priority in your life you will be a fitness role model even if—perhaps, more important, *because*—your child has special needs.

Of course, the effort it takes for you to accomplish a workout might require special needs all your own: where or when you can work out might be limited, and finding appropriate child care might be more challenging. Because taking care of your child is that much more demanding, the need to take care of yourself is that much greater. In addition to the mental break a workout might bring, moms with special needs children often need a greater degree of physical strength to manage lifting, moving, and carrying a growing child.

Many people are familiar with Team Hoyt, the father/son duo of Dick and Rick Hoyt (http://www.teamhoyt.com). Rick was born quadriplegic with cerebral palsy. His father, a runner and triathlete, has trained and raced with Rick since their first five-mile run together in 1977. The number of finish lines they have crossed are too numerous to count and their inspiration to all parents too much to quantify. In order to bring fitness to your child and get workouts in together, you don't have to pull your child on a raft while swimming 2.4 miles, then cycle 112 miles on a modified bike, and follow that up with a marathon pushing a wheelchair like Dick, but he certainly proves that anything is possible.

Like any mom, you have to look for opportunities and situations that can accommodate a workout. The strategies might encompass any of those mentioned for the above ages and stages, or you might need to devise tactics of your own. For instance, if your child is in physical or occupational therapy—often a workout in its own right—use that time to move yourself. Remember the characteristics that increase your odds of getting in a workout back in chapter 6: Adaptability, initiative, confidence, persistence, and creativity are integral to being a fit mom.

Another role you may have the privilege of participating in is that of "guide." For instance, children with sight impairments need a partner to "illustrate" the terrain or give directions. Blind cyclists typically ride tandem with a sighted partner, and visually impaired runners often run tethered to a sighted partner. If you are a mother taking on this role then you are opening yourself up to a unique and gratifying experience. And no doubt, by pushing the boundaries of your child's ability, you are giving your child a unique and gratifying experience, as well.

There are many organizations created for the sole purpose of supporting people in their specific disabilities. Tap into these resources for guidance and support for modifying exercise appropriately. (Or maybe, as a fit mom, you can lead the charge!) One organization dedicated to helping athletes pursue an active lifestyle is the Challenged Athletes Foundation (http://www.challengedathletes.org), which raises money to provide grants for special sporting equipment for people with disabilities.

Blending Ages and Abilities

Most parents have to find a way to incorporate fitness into a family with different ages and abilities. Many of these strategies can work with various ages, and some can even be doubled up (for example, run with one child in a jogger as an older child rides alongside on his bike).

Because your goal is also to expose your kids to fitness (and to enjoy it enough so you can work out, too) take some time on the front end to organize these workouts.

■ Find activities that suit various ages, abilities, and fitness levels.

■ Adapt activities for younger or special needs children so that everyone feels satisfied.

■ Let kids take turns picking out which activity they want to do (because when do siblings ever agree?).

It's one thing to be a fit mom, but to teach your children the value of fitness and to raise a fit family as well is infinitely more rewarding—not to mention impressive. That's why you're a role model not only to your children, but to other moms as well.

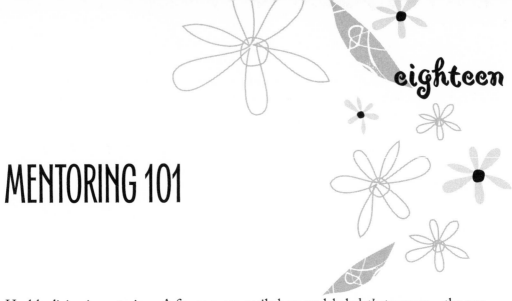

eighteen

MENTORING 101

Healthy living is contagious. A fit mom can easily become labeled *that* woman—the one who seems to effortlessly juggle all those balls, whose body exudes health, and who still has the energy to smile. Her light becomes a beacon. People will ask: How do you do it? Sure, underneath it all you might still feel a little crazed, but regardless you hold something of value they may want and need. That light is your fitness, and fit moms should be prepared to share their light, and if they're inclined, help others succeed, too.

Who, Me?

Sometimes we step into the role of mentor intentionally, in hopes to inspire a sister, mother, or friend. Perhaps we're asked, and our mentoring relationship is acknowledged and discussed openly. At other times we may be unaware or merely suspect we play the role we do. Friends who always assumed running a 5K was beyond their reach find themselves registering for a race or setting a goal they never thought possible. From you they begin to see they can be both mother and athlete.

There are other times we act as mentors and we don't even know it. Women at work, at the gym, and at the park will see what you do and be inspired. No, you may never know the impact you have on these women, but your lifestyle gives them a sense of hope they didn't have before.

Now don't be so humble; it's true, other women look up to you. Maybe you're not the fittest mom, or the most "put together" mom, or even the happiest mom on the block, but you show the world what really matters by how you live your life. You've not given up on yourself. You haven't lost touch with yourself as an individual. And while life might not always go as planned, you're constantly trying, which makes you both human and admirable. The choice to be admired by others isn't always yours to make. Other women will naturally look to you for support in their quest for fitness.

What Kids Think About Their Fit Moms

Whether or not you actively mentor another mom, be sure in the fact that you're making an impact on your kids. These moms have kids who notice.

- My kids are proud of me and every once in a while they ask me to "flex" for one of their friends.
- My five-month-old was unresponsive when I asked her what she thought of my fitness. But I am sure she was thinking she can't wait for me to start running so she can run with me.
- My girls are only thirteen months old, but I think that my exercise routine has helped them learn how to count since I count reps out loud!
- Sometimes they are frustrated when I leave to work out, but they love when I bring home a medal or they attend an event and have fun.
- My little boys just wonder why I am so "yucky" when I get home.
- They think I am crazy for getting up so early in the morning!
- They like that I win races! (Disclaimer: I have never won a race, but they think if I get a medal that I won!)
- I've heard my sons tell their friends that I run. My eight-year-old told his class, "My mom ran that marathon on her fortieth birthday and got like in the top ten!" It was actually more like the lower third, but I love to be on his top ten list!
- They dig having a mom who can ski with them and basically keep up. They tell me they are proud of me.
- My kids think everyone works out as much I do. They are always showing me their "muscles" and telling me that when they grow up they are going to beat me in all the races.
- They wonder why I look so tired and have a red face when I am done!
- They love the fact that Mom is strong and can flip tires and push Jeeps. They love to give me a hug even when I am all sweaty!

- My son will ask me, "Mom, did you go run today?" If I say no, he will ask me "Why not?" If I say yes, it's "How far?" Talk about accountability!
- A few months after giving birth to my third baby, my three-year-old came up to me and patted my belly and said, "Mom, you really need to start exercising again."
- They told me my forty-mile bike ride last weekend was "epic." But in general, they take it for granted. I support their pursuits, and they support mine. It's just what we do.

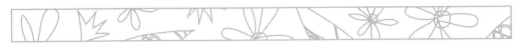

We all look up to fit women, but fit *moms* deserve special recognition. And the key to being a fit mama mentor is to never forget the mama part. As you know by now, it's important to model a healthy lifestyle to your kids. You don't pursue fitness at the expense of your kids—sometimes you reshape your workouts to include them, sometimes you push or pull them to keep them at your side, other times you forgo exercise to keep life sane. Those who manage the duties of motherhood along with their need to get and stay in shape put forth extra effort, determination, and perseverance.

But being a fit-mom mentor isn't the same as being a personal trainer. No, you're much more than just a trainer; you are an empowering source of inspiration, a life-changing (not just a body-changing) influence. Sure, you can help people achieve their fitness goals, but the first step is modeling and suggesting ways for others to feel nourished by fitness, instead of stressed by it. Heck, we all still need that reminder now and then.

So while it's great to help others achieve their fitness goals, you cannot be responsible for another human being. You can't do the work for them and you can't bear their discontent, either. True, without you to look up to some moms might not remember they deserve the time to get fit, but ultimately you're not responsible for getting them out the door. There's a fine line between mentoring and codependence. Remember those priorities we talked about way back in chapter 1? Stick to them

Who's Your Mommy (Mentor)?

Most of us who have the mojo to motivate other moms have our own source of inspiration to get moving. Here's what some women had to say about the fit moms who inspire them.

Around Every Corner

- Any woman who can give me hope is my mom mentor.
- My next-door neighbor inspired me to "do it anyway." She didn't know she was providing the example I needed.
- I have a friend whose life is more hectic than mine and she still makes time. She has shown me that achieving her goals and the health (mental and physical) benefits of exercise has made her a better wife and mother.
- That bitch has abs of steel!
- There is a lady at my gym who has cancer. I saw her all the time while I was pregnant. When I came back after my maternity leave she was bald as a cue ball from her cancer treatments. She is a group cycling instructor and has not stopped doing this throughout treatment. I barely even know her name, but she helped me realize that you can make time to work out for your mental and physical well-being no matter what personal challenges you may have. She has three kids and the most positive attitude of any cancer patient I have ever encountered. She credits a lot of her success to being fit while fighting. She is a true inspiration.
- My sister is crazy fit with four kids. I figure if she can figure out a way to make it happen, so can I.
- All of my running girlfriends are my fit-mom mentors. They remind me to be fit not frumpy!
- An instructor at my gym encouraged me. Seeing her do all that she did before 6 a.m. with three kids at home made me know I could do it, too. She never made excuses for me but taught me not to be so hard on myself.
- The "old me" is my inspiration. Before I remarried, I was a single mom of one. I managed to work full-time, go to school, be a mom, and so on, and still fit in time to run. I turned forty and missed that sense of accomplishment, that I could do something hard (as if the rest of my life wasn't hard at the time). So I bought a pair of shoes and took off. I haven't looked back.

- One of my yoga instructors has two small children but is fit as can be. She is so lively and I know it's partly because she's fit and has energy.
- I aspire to be a mentor—for someone else.

The Moms Have It!

- My mom has always been active and energetic. She recently survived cancer and still manages to ride two horses, clean the barn, throw bales, and inline skates six miles daily. Did I mention she is seventy?
- My mother was always at the beach, playing volleyball, surfing, and riding bikes, and after all of that she would drag me to the gym!
- My mother-in-law was an amazing woman and was a great inspiration to me in many facets of my life, especially fitness. When I met her she was a breast cancer survivor with a tenacious spirit. Regardless of her peaks and valleys, both emotionally and physically, she always made time to exercise.
- My mother took the time to stay in shape her entire life and is extremely healthy now because of it.
- My mother understands how hard it is to fit in a workout. But she raised me (and my three siblings) to realize that it's essential to my well-being and that I shouldn't feel guilty about it. She always encourages me to keep going and buys me cute workout gear on my birthday.
- My mother was and still is a fit mom. She is turning eighty this year and still walks and plays tennis and golf. I have memories of her doing Jane Fonda workouts in the living room while I did my homework, going out for a cross-country ski on my snow days, and always heading out for an hour-long walk whenever she could. She jogged until she was about fifty and started doing yoga when she was sixty-eight! I've learned to take care of my body and mind through exercise, and I hope I am in as great shape as she is when I am her age.
- My mom is a great mentor to me. She has been working out since I was a teen and while I didn't see the importance then, I do now. I look to her for guidance regarding my health and fitness.

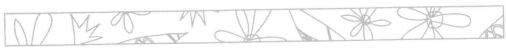

So, What Do I Do Now?

Sharing what you know with enthusiasm goes a long way toward helping others achieve their goals. But there are a few other things you can do to encourage and inspire without too much hand-holding. Here are six things you can do to help other moms get hot and sweaty. They are the keys to being an effective MENTOR.

Motivate
Explain
Nurture
Target
Orchestrate
Respond

Motivate

Start by determining what is motivating this mom to get fit. If she starts with a goal of weight loss, help her dig a little deeper to discover the real, underlying motivation. Is it health? Sanity? Competition? Independence? All of the above? Knowing this will help you offer better-directed encouragement and provide words that elicit positive emotional and physical responses.

Explain

Being a fit mom is all about choices. We make choices on a daily basis regarding time management, diet, and exercise. The choices we make must be congruent with our fitness goals, lifestyle, and, most important, our values. Understanding that the choice is her responsibility to make will make the transition from mom to fit mom easier. Explain this with words and in action.

Nurture

Teach her to be honest with herself and to set realistic expectations. Understand that there will be days and weeks when the workouts will be effortless and you will have a lot more time to work out than not. Conversely there will be times when throwing in the towel may *seem* easier. Help her to build an attitude of perseverance and determination with encouragement and praise.

Target

Help her to set realistic and measurable goals and remind her that goal setting should take into account the seasons in her life. Then help her target a consistent amount of time to devote to fitness in order to reach that goal.

Orchestrate

You've got her on the path to life as a fit mom. Now is the time to orchestrate a workout or two together, invite her over for dinner to cook a healthy meal, or hit a nice restaurant to celebrate a month of sticking to her goals.

Respond

Respond to her efforts by offering feedback. People trying to attain a goal are more successful if they get reminders, gentle nudging, feedback, encouragement, and so on, regarding their efforts. A weekly phone call, text, or e-mail will help, as will being available to answer questions and offering helpful suggestions. Even an occasional snail-mail card that says "Go, Girl!" will provide loads of confidence.

No matter what type of mentoring relationship you are in, always allow for a long leash. Your friend should want her fitness more than you want her fitness. Remember, health is hers to gain or not. You already have yours.

When They Don't Take the Bait

You know how great it is to be fit; it's no wonder you want that for someone who is close to you, or someone who has asked you to help her achieve the same fit lifestyle you have. Sometimes, it turns out, she doesn't end up following through in the same way you did. Despite the fact that you watched her children so she could work out, let her borrow your heart-rate monitor so she could get a visual guideline (almost like sharing underwear, but not quite), offered to work out with her, and even entered a race together, this friend, who initially expressed interest in getting fit, just won't follow through. You've been turned down so many times you feel like a spurned lover.

At this point, your job is done. Feel good knowing you've planted the seeds of fit living. Take heart in knowing that that seed may sprout in the future, and then consider the following advice:

1. Don't take it personally. She's not "with you" or "against you." As you know, life comes with challenges, and she's got to figure out how to overcome them in order to get fit.

2. Continue to inquire about her fitness goals but not to excess; don't turn her off of fitness by hounding her too often.

3. Keep the friendship alive. If your friendship was healthy prior to this, then there's no reason it shouldn't be now. If this mentoring relationship put a strain on your friendship you might need to take a deep breath and return to your regular routine.

Sweet Success

More often, the outcome of your mentoring efforts will be the addition of a new friend or family member into the fit life. Very quickly, you will begin to learn things from your protégé. Perhaps she'll share new strategies for squeezing in a workout, or maybe she'll turn out to be a gifted athlete who shares training tips with you. It doesn't matter, really, because being fit is highly contagious. You'll have more support with each passing day, as new moms become Hot (Sweaty) Mamas right beside you.

You're a Hot (Sweaty) Mama Now

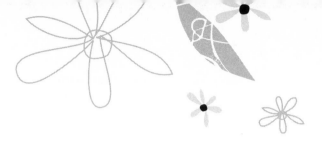

When did all these attempts to squeeze in exercise turn you into a fit mom? Over time, when you finally started to make it to more workouts than you had to miss, the metamorphosis began and without knowing exactly when it happened, you became a Hot (Sweaty) Mama.

By the way, you can't ever go back. Once a Hot (Sweaty) Mama, always a Hot (Sweaty) Mama. But wait, you think, what if I lapse and go through a two-month dry spell without a workout? We're counting on two things here: One, if you're not working out it's a conscious decision due to a temporary imbalance in your life, and you know you'll get back at it eventually. And, two, in that absence of fitness you still believe in its benefits, be it health, weight management, sanity, and so forth, and look forward to making exercise the conduit to these benefits once again.

Sure, being a Hot (Sweaty) Mama is about action, but it's also a state of mind. There will most definitely be times when finding the time and energy for a workout isn't a priority in your day. What matters most is that continuum in your life, that it's mostly steady with a few highs and lows. You've heard it before: Moms *can* have it all, just not necessarily all at the same time. Accepting this reality is essential to being a *happy* Hot (Sweaty) Mama.

Achieving Your Personal Best as a Fit Mom

As you travel along life's path, remember to look at the big picture. Keeping perspective is a valuable quality. Being realistic, a huge plus. Oh, and being forgiving is helpful, too. We know you understand that like the rest of life, fitness is a journey. We're always striving; always aspiring.

So now you know the five secrets to life as a fit mom. Before we end the book, however, we'll leave you with three more important action items.

1. **Set goals in accordance with your stage in life.** When planning a future that includes fitness, it's helpful to set unique goals that take into account the challenges of motherhood. The younger your children are the more difficult it will be to allocate large chunks of time to grandiose fitness goals. Sure it can be done now, but with a fair share of sacrifice. Know what kind of trade-offs you're willing to make.

2. **Set personal records for motherhood as well as for fitness.** Goal setting isn't limited to fitness. Set goals in your personal life. Determine what you want to do best in your world. What kind of accomplishments do you want to make as a mother?

3. **Grow old gracefully as a Hot (Sweaty) Mama.** There are no age limits. That's why it's important to take into account the big picture. The centenarian who walks every day? The eighty-five-year-old woman who skydives? The great-grandma who medals in three events at the Senior Olympics? Whoever she is, we want to grow up to be her. The focus isn't about having "the race of our lives"; instead we need to aim to race for the rest of our lives.

We're confident we're leaving you and your family more fit, if not by motivation, then with a few tools to pry open a small portion of your day to shove in a workout. Tending to our various roles, needs, and responsibilities while staying fit can give our lives an absurd, yet endearing, quality. At the end of the day, everything we can accomplish is both impressive and ridiculous at the same time.

And so what if it appears ridiculous? The shenanigans are all worth it in the quality of your life—which has now been extended, thanks to your making exercise a priority. You now have the confidence to feel worthy of a fit life. Show us your muscles. Show us your smile. Show us your fit family. How ridiculous is that?

Appendix

Fit Mom Supply List

We asked more than two hundred women what essentials they needed to be fit moms, and we added some of our own. You may not need everything listed here, but if it helps another mom out there find fitness in the chaos of motherhood, maybe it can help you, too.

Things That Make Her Go

- Energy drink
- Hydration drink
- Energy gels or chews for longer workouts
- Your own protein-shake recipe (Kara's favorite: Blend yogurt, frozen cherries, frozen pineapple, a splash of milk or buttermilk, and a scoop of protein powder)

Look Good/Feel Good

- All-day fitness attire
- Running skirts
- A good sports bra
- All things Dri-FIT
- Flip-flops/comfort shoes
- Cute hair accessories to keep hair and sweat out of your face

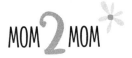

A Starbucks card! I often work at night to make up for hours missed in the middle of the day to work out, which means I sleep less and I have become quite a coffee drinker. Before kids, I never drank a drop!

—Karen, mom of two
San Jose, California

I love my Under Armour high-impact sports bra. I can even get it off when I am sweaty!

—Julie, mom of two
Bryan, Texas

Safety, Safety, Safety

- Personal identification
- Cell phone
- Pepper spray
- Reflective clothing
- Headlamp for night walks/runs

Good Gear That Makes Exercise Happen

- Resistance bands
- Exercise ball
- Dumbbells
- Yoga props (mat, block, belt)
- Bicycle
- Jump rope
- Ankle weights
- Removable pull-up bar
- Sport-specific gear (hockey stick, tennis racket, golf clubs, softball glove)

Good Gear That Makes Exercise with Kids Happen

- Jogging stroller
- Weather shield for stroller
- Bike trailer
- Attachable bike seat
- Bike "tagalong"
- A bike trainer that allows you to "spin" at home
- Treadmill
- Baby-containment devices (bouncy seat, swing, playpen)
- Backpack or front carrier (choose an option that supports the child's weight on your hips, as well as your shoulders)

MOM 2 MOM

A garage that locks so no one steals your jogging stroller, which happened to me and it totally ruined my training momentum, not to mention bumming me and my kids out big time!

—Patty, mom of two
Minneapolis, Minnesota

A visualization board to post your goals, inspirational quotes, and/or pictures to keep yourself focused on your ultimate goal!

—Sharon, mom of two
San Antonio, Texas

MOM 2 MOM

I make my own do-it-yourself baby wraps (search http://wearyourbaby.com). I spent eight dollars on fabric and made two. I go on so many walks with my baby!

—Anne, mom of one
Woburn, Massachusetts

- Laundry basket filled with toys for impromptu visits to the track, park, tennis court, and so on
- Wheels for the kids (bike, scooter, inline skates) that allow them to roll with you on a walk, run or ride

Good Gear That Enhances the Exercise Experience

- Water bottle/carrier (backpack or belt)
- Sports watch and/or heart-rate monitor
- Armband holder for music player
- Good earphones that don't fall out
- Exercise journal/log (Joanne, mom of two in Saskatoon, Saskatchewan, e-mails herself the details of her workout for her online fitness journal)
- Sunglasses
- Sunscreen (don't forget the kiddos!)
- Stretching and self-massage accessories (straps, balls, plastic and foam rollers ... hurts so good!)
- Compression sleeves

Good Places/Services That Support the Fit Mom

- Gym membership with child care
- Fit mom exercise classes
- A good local running store to help properly fit your shoes
- A good local bike shop to ensure proper bike fit/setup

People That Can Help Take Care of Mom

- A doctor that "gets you" (Getting the all-clear before starting to exercise, if you've never worked out or haven't in a long while, is highly recommended. Having a medical expert in your camp when you're sidelined with illness or injury is convenient—possibly even a lifesaver.)
- A good chiropractor

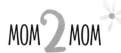

MOM 2 MOM

Get a good planner. Doesn't matter if it's electronic, a wall calendar, or an old notebook. If you don't schedule your workouts and make them a priority in your day, you will never get it done.

—Tonia, mom of three
Glen Allen, Virginia

- Massage therapist
- Flexible babysitters
- Grandparents who live nearby (Laurie is forever grateful to Grandpa Tony, who lives just a few blocks away and often makes her workouts possible.)
- A personal trainer or an online coach
- Sisters in sweat! ("A group of fit moms helps you to keep coming up with new ideas as the kids change," says Stephanie, mom of two in San Jose, California.)

Intangibles
- Goals
- Confidence
- Courage
- Determination
- A smile ("I always work out better when I'm in a good mood," says Samantha, mom of two in Torrance, California.)

MOM 2 MOM

Sex with a great partner!

—Tricia, mom of one
Pittsburgh, Pennsylvania

A BFAW (best friend at work) who will ask about your latest workout or next event.

—Paula, mom of two
Chanhassen, Minnesota

Resources

Thanks to a "fit-mom survey" we conducted (see page 195 for a summary), two-hundred-plus fit moms helped us compile a list of resources that support the fit life. Here's what helps other moms stay fit.

Books

- *Run Like a Mother: How to Get Moving and Not Lose Your Job, Family, or Sanity*, by Dimity McDowell and Sarah Bowen Shea (Andrews McMeel Publishing, 2010)
- *Exercising Through Your Pregnancy*, by James Clapp (Addicus Books, 2002)
- *Fit Pregnancy for Dummies*, by Catherine Cram and Tere Stouffer Drenth (Wiley, 2004)
- *Female Body Breakthrough: The Revolutionary Strength-Training Plan for Losing Fat and Getting the Body You Want*, by Rachel Cosgrove (Rodale Books, 2009)
- *Gold Medal Fitness: A Revolutionary Five-Week Program*, by Dara Torres (Broadway Books, 2010)
- *Yoga: The Iyengar Way*, by Silva Mehta, Mira Mehta, and Shyam Mehta (Knopf, 1990)
- *Chi Running: A Revolutionary Approach to Effortless, Injury-Free Running*, by Danny Dreyer and Katherine Dreyer (Fireside, 2009)
- *Slow, Fat Triathlete: Live Your Athletic Dreams in the Body You Have Now*, by Jayne Williams (Marlowe and Company, 2004)
- *Triathlons for Women*, by Sally Edwards (VeloPress, 2010)
- *The Heart Rate Guidebook to Heart Zones Training*, by Sally Edwards (Heart Zones Publishing, 2010)

DVDs

- *Jillian Michaels 30-Day Shred* ("It's only twenty minutes long! We can all find twenty minutes to work out each day," says Heather, mom of two in Toronto, Canada.)
- *Lose Your Mummy Tummy* with Julie Tupler
- P90X home fitness training system
- The Firm series of workouts
- *OM Yoga* with Cyndi Lee
- *Yoga Conditioning for Athletes* with Rodney Yee
- *Spinervals* with Troy Jacobson

- *Aligned and Well* by Katy Bowman, (which includes the *Down There for Women* DVD for strengthening the pelvic floor)
- 10 Minute Solution series of workouts
- Windsor Pilates series of workouts

Websites
- http://www.hotsweatymamas.com
- http://www.mapmyrun.com
- http://www.active.com
- http://www.gotribalnow.com
- http://www.dailymile.com
- http://www.fitness.com
- http://www.livestrong.com
- http://www.lifeasafitmom.com
- http://www.seemommyrun.com
- http://www.momsinmotion.com
- http://www.onefamilyonemeal.com (This chef and mother of two provides a weekly meal menu with recipes and a shopping list—she aims to spend less than two hundred dollars for mostly organic and natural products—to make dinner easy and enjoyable for a busy mom and finicky kids.)
- http://www.realfoodmoms.com

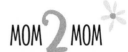

Self.com has videos of someone demonstrating exercise moves, which can be difficult to understand in a magazine.

—Kayris, mom of two
Baltimore, Maryland

Our Blogs
- http://www.mamasweat.blogspot.com (Kara's blog on finding fitness in the chaos of motherhood)
- http://www.seemomsweat.blogspot.com (Laurie's blog on balancing motherhood and fitness)

Twenty-Eight-Day Fitness Challenge

Give us twenty-eight days (c'mon, it's like one menstrual cycle) and we'll show you what it's like to live a fit lifestyle. Here's how to carve out your week for exercise so that you can develop the fitness habit. You'll notice we're not telling you what specific exercises you should do; that's for you to decide. If you need some direction, look back to chapter 8 ("Get Moving") or chapters 16 and 17 ("Joined at the Hip" and "Child's Play") for more about how you should spend your exercise time and how to exercise with kids present. Be sure to write your workouts down in your calendar or exercise log so you can see what you've accomplished and track your progress.

Week 1

Set This in Stone: Schedule one workout that gets your heart rate going for *at least* thirty minutes. Make this cardio workout nonnegotiable.

Strength/Stretch: Take another workout this week to focus on strengthening and stretching muscles. Options here might include getting to a Pilates class, checking out a yoga book with illustrations that you can follow, or lifting milk jugs in your kitchen and lunging down the hallway.

Pep Talk: If your workouts are thirty minutes each session, that's only one hour of your week you need to carve out for fitness. You can handle this! If you're feeling overwhelmed, just take it one workout at a time and tell yourself it's only thirty minutes. In the words of René Descartes: "Divide each difficulty into as many parts as is feasible and necessary to resolve it."

Reward: You exercised two times this week! If you weren't exercising at all before that's quite a leap. Even for occasional exercisers, that suggests a commitment to fitness is in the works. At the beginning of the week determine how you will reward yourself for accomplishing week one—something small (it's been only one week, after all) but indulgent nonetheless. Download some new tunes to pump you up for the next week or buy something for your "active" wardrobe. At a minimum, acknowledge this success by being *proud* of yourself.

Week 2

Set This in Stone: Bump up to two thirty-minute cardio workouts this week. If the day and time you chose for last week worked well, stick with that and find one more thirty-minute slot. Experiment with days and times so that your nonnegotiable workouts work for you.

Strength/Stretch: At least one more workout should focus on strengthening and stretching muscles. You can always tack this workout to the beginning or end of a cardio workout.

Bonus: If time allows, lengthen one or more of these three workouts by five or ten minutes.

Pep Talk: You are now working out three times a week! The longer your workouts are, the better off your brain is at manufacturing those "feel-good" hormones. That said, even if you have only twenty minutes to devote to exercise, we believe that you're better off with a little exercise than none at all. Make sure you write even these "baby steps" toward fitness down in your calendar/exercise log. Continue to plug away: As Winston Churchill said, "Success is not final, failure is not fatal: It is the courage to continue that counts."

Reward: You're halfway through. While fitness might not feel like a habit just yet, you have lived two whole weeks with a fit lifestyle. Go ahead, brag about it. Call someone and tell them about this new change in your life.

Week 3

Set This in Stone: Continue with two nonnegotiable cardio workouts for *at least* forty-five minutes. Again, make sure these nonnegotiable workouts "sync" with your schedule. If not, find better days/times. This is crucial to making these workouts nonnegotiable.

Strength/Stretch: At least one thirty-minute workout this week should focus on strengthening and stretching muscles. Remember the creative ways to squeeze this into your day if you have to (triceps dips on the side of the bathtub, stretching while you play with blocks, and so on).

Bonus: Can you find one more thirty-minute slot in the week to work out?

Pep Talk: You're still working out three times a week, but have added a half hour (or more if you're on the bonus plan) to your weekly exercise time. Don't be overwhelmed. In the grand scheme of things, you're required to find only two hours for fitness each week. But don't look at the whole; break it up into its smaller pieces, remember? As your body gets stronger, so does your mind. "Strength does not come from physical capacity. It comes from an indomitable will," said Mahatma Gandhi.

Reward: You've just rewarded yourself with twenty-one days of fit living. Go take a look in the mirror. What do you see? You may or may not notice the physical rewards of exercise yet, but we're certain you're standing straighter and holding your chin a little higher. Now smile and thank that woman in the mirror.

Week 4

Set This in Stone: Three forty-five-minute workouts (two for cardio). By now you should have an arrangement that you can hang on to. This is your base. When all else fails, you still get a minimum of three workouts each week.

Strength/Stretch: At least one of these workouts should focus on strengthening and stretching muscles.

Bonus: Can you increase your three workouts to one hour each, or add in one more forty-five-minute session? That's just forty-five more minutes in the 10,080 minutes you have each week.

Pep Talk: This week is all about maintaining your workouts—giving you confidence that you can, indeed, live this fit lifestyle. No, you may not always get three workouts in each week. Yes, sometimes you will exercise for a shorter period of time than you intended, but as Ralph Waldo Emerson says, "We aim above the mark to hit the mark."

Reward: The only worthy reward you can give yourself is making the decision to carry on with your new habit!

Beyond the Next Twenty-Eight Days

Three thirty-minute workouts is the minimum of fitness we aim for; the ideal is an hour of exercise on most days of the week. Spend the next month clinging to your thrice-weekly workout schedule. Once that feels part of your groove, start adding workouts where it makes sense, in whatever ways you can: Make time, take time, share time, snare time. Some weeks you might find you can work out five times; other weeks you can squeeze it in only twice. This is the ebb and flow of a fit life. Remember, though: Don't get caught up in what you can't do; celebrate what you can.

Fit Mom Inventory and Examples

Are your perceived priorities in line with your actual priorities? It's time to take inventory on your life. What is it you value most? How do these values translate into priorities? How do these priorities guide your day?

1. Make a list of your values. Before you Google "values," which is what we did, spend a few minutes thinking about what genuinely matters to you, and make sure you include those values that were important to you before you had children. You don't want the list to be too long; narrow your values to the most cherished: Make a list of ten or less. If you're satisfied with your list move on to the next step, but if you feel there's another value or two underneath the surface that you can't put your finger on, then turn to the Internet to help you clarify the ones that are important to you. Here's a short list:

achievement	family	integrity	privacy
ambition	financial stability	intelligence	respect
charity	fitness	learning	trust
cleanliness	friendship	liberty	vitality
creativity	happiness	love	wisdom
excellence	health	order	
faith	honesty	philanthropy	

2. Record your daily activities. Grab a notebook and spend a day or two tracking what you do with your time. Make sure it's a typical day—don't bother doing this when you're on vacation or Grandma is in town to lend an extra hand. There's no need for elaborate entries, either; just jot down a list of where and how you're spending your time throughout the day.

3. Create categories for your actions (for example, career, mommy chores, family time, philanthropy, personal enrichment, fitness, and so on).

4. Now, return to your list of values and, when possible, assign a value to each category. If one of your categories doesn't correspond with a value, leave it blank. The fewer blank slots you have, the better you are at spending time in a way that resonates with your values.

5. List in ascending order those values that get your most time and attention. Whether you like it or not, where you allot the most time translates into your actual priorities. Take note here: Are your *perceived priorities* in line with your *actual priorities*?

Laurie's Sample Inventory
May 21, 2010

Time Tracker	Activity	Category	Corresponding Value
5:00–7:00 a.m.	cup of coffee and off to teach group cycling class	exercise socializing	health/fitness friendship
7:00–8:00 a.m.	breakfast and coffee with family, make lunches	family time nutrition	family health/fitness
8:00–8:30 a.m.	take kids to school and preschool	kid duties kid time	family
8:30–9:30 a.m.	practice yoga	exercise	health/fitness spirituality
9:30–10:45 a.m.	shower, get dressed, do breakfast dishes, vacuum, clean up a bit	hygiene household chores	self-care family
10:45 a.m. –noon	therapy	mental health	self-care spirituality
Noon–2 p.m.	meet neighbor and preschoolers (she picked them up today) at the park for picnic and play	friendship kid time play	friends family fun/adventure
2:00–2:30 p.m.	pick up grade schooler, talk with other parents, head home	kid time friendship	family friends
2:30–3:30 p.m.	get snacks for kids, homework for older daughter, read and/or TV time for kids, e-mail and phone calls for me	kid chores nutrition work	family health/fitness learning/intellectual
3:30–5:30 p.m.	kids play outside with neighbors, I start dinner, practice guitar, read and do some writing out front	reading music career	spirituality learning/intellectual
5:30–6:30 p.m.	eat dinner and make cookies with family	nutrition family time baking	health/fitness family fun/adventure
6:30–7:00 p.m.	walk the dogs with husband and kids	family time exercise	family health/fitness spirituality
7:00–7:30 p.m.	do dishes while husband gives the kids a bath and gets them ready for bed	household chores	family
7:30–8:00 p.m.	eat cookies and watch something on Animal Planet (the kids love *Monsters Inside Me*!)	family time educational entertainment	family learning/intellectual fun/adventure
8:00–8:30 p.m.	get kids ready for and into bed, take kids back to bed, tell kids to get back into bed	kid duties	family
8:30–9:30 p.m.	read and watch television with husband	husband time relaxing	family self-care
9:30 p.m.	wash up, brush teeth, and head to bed with husband, "enjoy" the company of my husband	hygiene husband sexuality	self-care family health/fitness

Laurie's Values List	Actual Values Ranking
family	family (eleven entries)
friends	health/fitness (seven entries)
fun/adventure	spirituality (four entries)
learning/intellectual	self-care (four entries)
health/fitness	fun/adventure (three entries)
spirituality	learning/intellectual (three entries)
self-care	friends (two entries)

Developing my list of values was a fairly straightforward task for me. I'm happy to (finally!) be at a place in my life where I'm consciously making efforts to include all of my values and priorities in my daily life. I've worked hard to find a good schedule that allows me to exercise without much trouble. Teaching a morning group cycling class has been a twice-weekly activity for me for the past ten years. Getting up that early was a little more challenging when I was nursing and had to pump before I left, but even that became routine. Now, when I get home everyone is just rolling out of bed.

While family and fitness have always been no-brainers, spirituality was something I'd really lost sight of in the chaos of daily life. If I did this exercise a year ago, I might have had a zero for that category. I've learned that, for me, therapy, yoga, and music are all ways to develop myself spiritually. I was surprised to see that friends fell lower on my list, but I've made a choice to focus on myself a little more right now, so I guess it makes sense. Fun was a little ambiguous for me since I try to find fun in most things I do. The second part of that category, adventure, seems to have eluded me, though. I plan to work on making sure I have more adventure in my life. For the most part, this exercise reaffirmed my current lifestyle. Right now, I want to add something a little crazy to my days to make sure I experience and teach my girls a spirit of adventure.

Kara's Sample Inventory
May 28, 2010

Time Tracker	Activity	Category	Corresponding Value
5:30–7:00 a.m.	writing time: finish and send story to editor	career	creativity financial security
7:00–8:30 a.m.	breakfast with kids, getting dressed, morning routine	meal making mommy chores	health/fitness family
8:30–9:00 a.m.	talk to Mom on phone	family time	family
9:00–11:30 a.m.	go to gym with kids	fitness	health/fitness
11:30–1:00 p.m.	make/eat/clean up lunch, get twins on bus, baby in bed for nap, welcome preschool friend over for playdate	meal making mommy chores	health/fitness family
1:00–3:00 p.m.	start laundry, make appointment for wellness checkup, call insurance company about claim, catch up on e-mail and Facebook, start blog post	mommy chores friendship career	family friendship creativity
3:00–3:30 p.m.	baby up, play, draw chalk art on driveway with preschoolers, snack time	family time mommy chores	family creativity
3:30–4:30 p.m.	walk to park, playdate leaves, twins come home from school	family time fitness	family health/fitness
4:30–5:00 p.m.	more snacks, school debriefing	mommy chores family	family
5:00–6:30 p.m.	move clean laundry to pile on bed, start dinner, check on girls outside, talk to next-door neighbor, send e-mails to set up interviews for next article assignment, and finish dinner while baby plays with pots and pans	friendship career meal making	friendship financial security health/fitness
6:30–7:00 p.m.	eat dinner	family time	family
7:00–7:30 p.m.	bath for baby and put to bed	mommy chores	family
7:30–8:30 p.m.	husband home (quick smooch), call girls in, start bath, start folding clothes on bed, bedtime routine for girls	family time mommy chores	family
8:30–9:30 p.m.	intercept children getting out of bed, discard unfolded clothes to pile on floor, get ready for bed, watch mindless television with husband, crash	mommy chores unwind time family time	family (It's a stretch to call watching TV in the same room family time, but I'm going with it!)

Kara's Values List	Actual Values Ranking
creativity	family (eleven entries)
faith	health/fitness (five entries)
family	creativity (three entries)
financial security	financial security (two entries)
friendship	friendship (two entries)
health/fitness	faith (zero entries)

Considering I stay home with my kids, I expect family to be a top value with my time. I also lump time with extended family and my husband here, even though I know it's the kids who monopolize this category. I included the health/fitness value when I took time to prepare a meal because choosing to spend time making healthy food to eat aligns with health for me. While doing this exercise, I was surprised that financial security came up as a value for me. On the surface I like to think that money doesn't matter, and while I sincerely believe money doesn't buy happiness, I still have a need to be financially stable. I'm a little embarrassed I included faith as a value but didn't have a single corresponding activity! I might benefit from a few early morning moments in meditation. There are some days, though, when faith is more present or omnipresent (like during a solitary morning run while the sun rises). I believe, like my marriage, my faith is grounded from the "early work" and will survive with a drought here and there, whereas the needy young tendrils that are my children require constant care and watering. However, because these two things are important to me, I need to seek out ways to keep them more present in my day. In general, though, I was pleased with how my values translated into priorities and how my priorities guided my day.

Sweaty Decision Tree

There are times when skipping a workout makes sense; other times, you may need to talk yourself into working up that sweat. How do you know? It depends. To work out or not depends on your exercise habits in the days before and your plans in the days ahead. It depends on what will happen to your stress level if you do and if you don't. It depends on your feelings regarding missing a workout and, of course, your goals. We've designed a tree to factor all this in when you need help making that decision: Should I work out, or not?

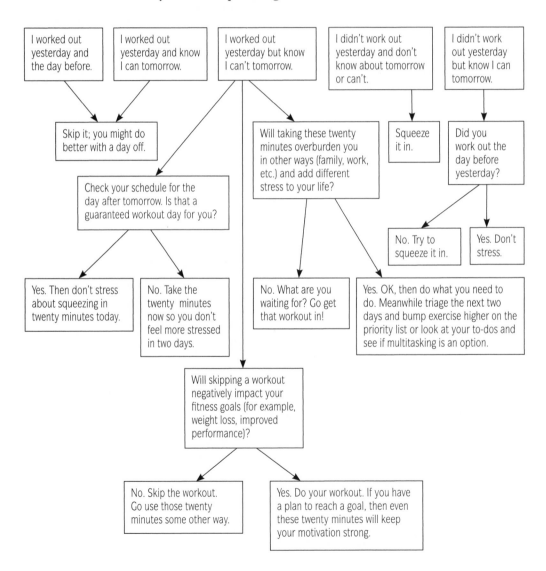

Fit Mom Survey

Additional insight into life as a fit mom was included in this book thanks to the help of more than two hundred fit moms who participated in our "Balancing Motherhood and Fitness" survey. Moms from all across the United States, Canada, Chile, France, Japan, New Zealand, and Portugal responded to our online survey, candidly communicating their stories of success and struggle in pursuit of the fit life. The stories and examples these women shared were more than fodder for this book; they are an inspiration for every mother and every future mother who wants to take charge of her life. Here we've condensed what they had to share.

Question 1: What's the craziest thing you've ever done to squeeze a workout into your already hectic day as a mom?

We've gotta hand it to these moms, they certainly are a creative lot. For this question, moms reported crazy activities that bordered on masochistic, and in some cases a little dangerous. Among the most popular: getting up in the wee hours of the morning, turning chores into workouts, and using children as exercise equipment. Check out "The Rise of the Hot (Sweaty) Mama" on page 1 for some of our favorites.

Question 2: Beyond weight goals, needing "me time," or health reasons, why is it important for you to exercise?

As you saw in the "Why Do You Exercise?" sidebar in chapter 2, some of the most popular reasons fit moms exercise include stress reduction, social time with workout partners, modeling healthy behavior to the kids, and alleviating depression. We listed some of the more unique reasons in the sidebar. You didn't miss them, did you?

Question 3: Have you ever felt guilty about choosing to work out versus do something else with your time? If yes, give us an example of what you felt you should have been doing instead.

Mother guilt is alive and kicking, isn't she? The majority, some 77 percent of our survey respondents, admitted that they have or do feel guilty when they choose to work out over some other task. The top guilt-inducing alternatives include spending time with the family and getting housework done. Spun more positively, 23 percent of our fit moms know they are worth the time. Kudos to you!

Question 4: Do you have or have you had a fit-mom mentor? (This could be anyone from Dara Torres to your next-door neighbor.) What was it about this fit mom that inspired you? How did she help you?

In chapter 18 you saw that virtually anyone can be a fit mama mentor (yes, that includes you!). Our moms listed everyone from a buff stranger at the gym, a cancer survivor, and a fitness instructor to (our favorite) their own moms.

Question 5: Does your partner/spouse support your pursuit of fitness?

Wow. Who knew support could be so helpful? We're happy to report 94 percent of our survey respondents said their spouse or partner supports their pursuit of fitness. Our hats off to the other 6 percent who make it work in the face of what can oftentimes be discouraging circumstances.

Question 6: What are some of your favorite workouts to do with kids in tow?

Depending on the age of their children, this question spawned a wide variety of responses from our fit mama respondents. Top picks for moms with younger kiddos were biking, walking, jogging, and yoga. Anything that wasn't already on our list made the book.

Question 7: If you don't end up doing the workout you planned, what is the number one reason (or excuse) that keeps you from it?

Tired and busy is how most moms describe themselves. No big surprise that these top two descriptors are Mom's biggest roadblock to fitness.

Question 8: What do your kids think about you working out? Don't know? Ask them and let us know what they say!

Chapter 18 has a list of some of the funnier responses we received. No bones about it, no matter what age our children are, they generally have something positive to say.

Question 9: We are building a "Fit Mom Supply List." Do you have any recommendation for essential gear, services, people, Web sites, books, videos, or other resources you need to help you be a fit mom?

This question drew so many great responses that we devoted an appendix section to it.